Sophia Harmon

SOMATIC EXERCISES
for Beginners

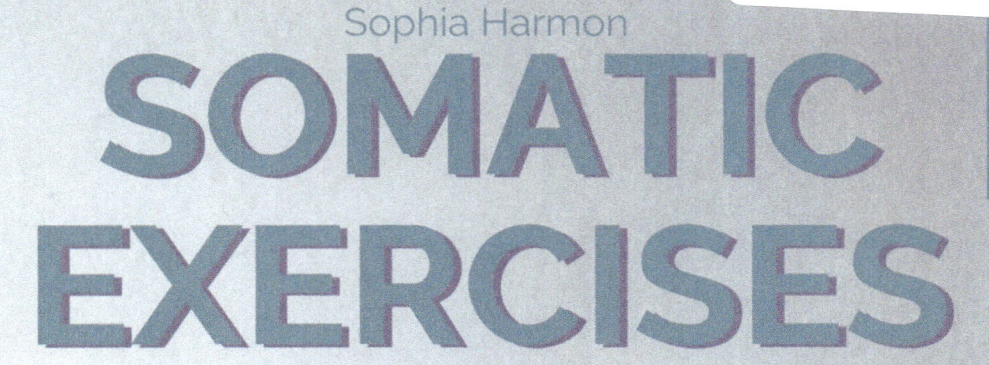

2024

EMOTIONAL BALANCE

WEIGHT LOSS

TENSION RELIEF

180+ REAL PHOTOS & 90 VIDEO TUTORIALS

3 BONUS COLORED EDITION

28-DAYS REVIVAL CHALLENGE

© **Copyright 2024 - All rights reserved.**

The contents of this book may not be reproduced, duplicated, or transmitted without the direct written permission of the author or publisher.

In no event will any fault or legal liability be held against the publisher or author for any damage, repair, or pecuniary loss due to the information contained in this book. Directly or indirectly.

Legal notice:

This book is copyrighted. This book is for personal use only. You may not modify, distribute, sell, use, quote, or paraphrase any part or content of this book without the consent of the author or publisher.

Notice of limitation of liability:

Please note that the information contained in this document is for educational and entertainment purposes only. Every effort has been made to present accurate, current, reliable, and complete information.

No warranty of any kind is stated or implied.

Readers acknowledge that the author does not undertake to provide legal, financial, medical, or professional advice. The content of this book has been derived from various sources. Please consult a licensed professional before attempting any of the techniques described in this book.

By reading this document, the reader agrees that in no event shall the author be liable for any loss, direct or indirect, incurred as a result of the use of the information contained in this document, including, but not limited to, errors, omissions, or inaccuracies.

TABLE OF CONTENTS

PART I: THEORETICAL FOUNDATIONS

1. INTRODUCTION TO SOMATIC EXERCISES

1.1 What are Somatic Exercises?	6
1.2 Benefits of Somatic Exercises	8
1.3 How Somatic Integrates into Daily Life	9

2. ESTABLISHING A SOMATIC EXERCISE ROUTINE

2.1 Creating a Personalized Routine	11
2.2 Maintaining Motivation and Monitoring Progress	13
2.3 Adaptations for Different Health Conditions	16

PART II: PRACTICAL EXERCISES

3. ANTI-STRESS EXERCISES

3.1 Exercises for Body Awareness (Grounding)	19
3.2 Exercises for Muscle Relaxation	22
3.3 Exercises for Chronic Pain	29
3.4 Exercises to Improve Mobility and Flexibility	32
3.5 Pre-Sleep Exercises	37

4. WARMING UP — 41

4.1 Mobility and Flexibility Exercises Pre-Workout	42
4.2 Muscle Awakening Exercises	47

5. MUSCLE STRENGTHENING EXERCISES

5.1 Basic Muscle Strengthening Exercises	52
5.2 Functional Exercises for Everyday Activities	55
5.3 Integration of Small Equipment	59
5.4 Weight Loss Exercises	62

6. 28-DAYS CHALLENGE — 67

Part I: Theoretical Foundations

Chapter 1: Introduction to Somatic Exercises

1.1 What are Somatic Exercises?

Definition
Somatic exercises are a form of **therapeutic** movement aimed at improving body awareness through the mindful exploration of movement. They emphasize the interaction between mind and body, helping to **relax** tense muscles and correct dysfunctional motor patterns. The primary goal is to reduce pain, increase **mobility** and flexibility, and improve overall well-being.

Origins and Historical Development
The practice of somatic exercises is based on the innovations of figures such as F.M. Alexander, Moshe Feldenkrais, and Thomas Hanna, who developed methods to improve physical function and mental well-being through greater body awareness.

- **F.M. Alexander**, an actor and acting teacher, developed the Alexander Technique in the early 20th century, an approach aimed at correcting harmful postural habits through increased awareness of body use. His techniques were based on the belief that better mental and physical coordination could resolve not only voice issues but also other physical disorders.
- **Moshe Feldenkrais**, an engineer and physicist, influenced by his own rehabilitation needs and interest in martial arts and biomechanics, introduced the Feldenkrais Method in the 1940s. This method emphasizes learning through movement and exploring new motor patterns to improve physical function and overall well-being.
- **Thomas Hanna**, a philosopher and somatic educator, integrated the principles of Alexander and Feldenkrais with modern discoveries in neurophysiology and motor control in the late 20th century, founding the discipline called Somatics. Hanna developed an educational approach that helped individuals recognize and modify their patterns of chronic tension through self-awareness and movement.

Throughout the 20th century, these methods merged into what we now know as somatic exercises, integrating principles of self-awareness, functional movement, and neurophysiology.

Fundamental Principles

The fundamental principles of somatic exercises are deeply rooted in understanding the interaction between mind and body and include:

1. **Body Awareness:** This principle is based on the idea that increased awareness of one's body can improve how we move and perceive physical sensations. Somatic exercises help individuals become more aware of their physical conditions, such as muscle tension and relaxation, and how these conditions affect their overall well-being. Self-awareness is developed through exercises that require attention and reflection on the sensations that emerge during movement.

2. **Muscle Relaxation:** Many physical problems and discomforts are caused or exacerbated by chronic muscle tension. Somatic exercises aim to identify and relax these tense muscles, allowing the body to release accumulated stress and pain. This is achieved through slow and controlled movements that enhance the ability to distinguish between necessary and unnecessary tension.

3. **Intentional Movement:** At the heart of somatic exercises is the intention with which each movement is performed. This principle emphasizes the importance of moving with awareness and deliberation rather than allowing the body to follow habitual patterns that may be harmful. Intentional and conscious movements help establish new patterns that are healthier and more effective, improving the overall quality of movement.

4. **Holistic Integration:** Somatic exercises do not focus solely on isolated body parts but seek to improve overall well-being through the integration of mind, body, and spirit. This holistic approach recognizes that physical well-being is intrinsically linked to mental and emotional health.

5. **Adaptability and Personalization:** Since every body is unique, somatic exercises emphasize the need to adapt and personalize exercises to meet the specific needs of each individual. This ensures that each movement maximizes benefits, ensuring the exercises are both safe and effective for everyone.

6. **Continuous Feedback:** Somatic learning is based on a continuous feedback loop between mind and body. The exercises are designed to increase the ability to perceive and respond to internal signals, facilitating progressive learning that adapts and evolves with individual experience.

Through these principles, somatic exercises offer a path towards a more integrated and conscious existence, where movement is not just a physical activity but becomes a means to discover and influence one's health and well-being on deeper levels.

1.2 Benefits of Somatic Exercises

Somatic exercises, characterized by their focus on body awareness and intentional movement, offer a wide range of benefits that can significantly improve individuals' quality of life. Among the most notable benefits are improved flexibility and mobility, reduced chronic pain, and effective stress and anxiety management.

Improvement in Flexibility and Mobility
Flexibility and mobility are essential for daily performance and maintaining a high level of physical functionality throughout life. Somatic exercises, through slow and controlled movements that increase body awareness, help release tension in muscles and joints. This muscle relaxation not only improves the range of motion but also the quality of each movement performed.
One mechanism through which somatic exercises improve mobility is neuromodulation, the process of retraining the central nervous system regarding muscle tone perception and regulation. Through repetitive practices emphasizing gentle and conscious movements, chronic tensions are released, allowing the body to regain its natural ability to move freely and painlessly.
Additionally, regular practice of somatic exercises increases the production of synovial fluid, the liquid that lubricates the joints, facilitating smoother movements and reducing the risk of injury. The benefits extend beyond the simple execution of exercises, positively influencing other daily activities, such as walking, sitting, and lifting objects, making these actions easier and less tiring.

Reduction of Chronic Pain
Chronic pain is a widespread condition affecting millions of people, often resulting from prolonged muscle tension, poor posture, and inefficient movements accumulated over time. Somatic exercises, by aiming to relax muscles and correct movement patterns, offer significant relief from these forms of pain.
Somatic practice helps individuals recognize and modify behaviors contributing to pain, such as poor postural habits or incorrect movements. By learning to identify early signs of tension and intervening through specific exercises, users can prevent pain from worsening and significantly increase their daily comfort.
A study showed that participants engaged in somatic exercises reported a 45% reduction in pain after only eight weeks of practice. This improvement in pain control is attributed to increased body awareness, enabling individuals to avoid movements and postures that exacerbate pain.

Stress and Anxiety Management

Stress and anxiety have a direct impact on physical and mental health, affecting everything from sleep quality to blood pressure. Somatic exercises are an effective tool for stress management due to their ability to calm the mind and relax the body.

Somatic practice encourages deep and controlled breathing, proven to lower cortisol levels, the stress hormone, and increase the production of endorphins, natural well-being chemicals. This process not only immediately reduces feelings of anxiety but also helps develop long-term resilience to stress.

Moreover, by focusing on movements and bodily sensations, somatic exercises promote a sense of presence and mindfulness, diverting attention from anxious or stressful thoughts. This mindfulness practice is often associated with mood improvements and reduced anxiety, making somatic exercises an effective complement to other forms of psychological and medical therapy for managing stress and anxiety.

In summary, somatic exercises offer profound and multidimensional benefits that extend beyond mere physical improvement. Through regular practice, individuals can not only enhance their flexibility and reduce pain but also acquire powerful tools for managing stress and improving their overall quality of life. These benefits make somatic exercises an ideal choice for anyone seeking to live a healthier, more active, and balanced life.

1.3 How Somatic Integrates into Daily Life

Somatic exercises, in addition to offering significant therapeutic benefits, can be easily integrated into daily life. This integration not only improves quality of life but also allows maintaining and amplifying the benefits obtained during formal practice. The following sections illustrate successful examples, the general impact on quality of life, and practical tips for incorporating somatic exercises into the daily routine.

Success Stories

Numerous case studies demonstrate the effectiveness of somatic exercises in bringing significant improvements to people's lives.
- Marie, a 45-year-old programmer, suffered from chronic back pain due to long hours spent sitting. After integrating somatic exercises into her daily routine, she not only experienced a significant improvement in pain but also increased her postural awareness, thus avoiding relapses in the long term.

- Luke, a middle school teacher, used somatic exercises to manage work-related stress. Through brief but regular daily practices, he noticed a significant reduction in stress levels and an improvement in his mood and ability to interact with students and colleagues.

Impact on Quality of Life

The integration of somatic exercises into daily life has a profound impact on quality of life. The benefits are manifold and vary from physical to emotional and psychological improvements. Regular practice can lead to reduced physical pain, increased flexibility and mobility, and better stress and anxiety management.

On a psychological level, the increased body awareness developed through somatic exercises can lead to improved self-perception and self-esteem. Individuals become more aware of their physical capabilities, which can translate into greater confidence in all areas of life.

Additionally, adopting somatic relaxation techniques can help improve sleep, reduce the risk of depression and anxiety, and even enhance interpersonal relationships due to a greater ability to manage emotional stress.

Tips for Integrating into Daily Routine

Integrating somatic exercises into the daily routine does not require radical changes or much time. Here are some practical tips for effectively incorporating these exercises:

- **Start the Day with Awareness:** Dedicating 5-10 minutes each morning to simple somatic exercises can help wake up the body and prepare it for the day's activities. Exercises like cat-cow or gentle torso twists can be done even in bed before getting up.
- **Active Breaks During Work:** For those who spend many hours sitting, it is beneficial to insert short somatic breaks every hour to stretch and relax the body. Small exercises like raising the arms, shoulder rotations, or neck stretches can be done even in limited spaces and help keep the body active and the mind clear.
- **Integration with Other Activities:** Somatic exercises can be combined with other forms of physical activity such as walking, swimming, or yoga. This not only makes the practice more varied and enjoyable but also helps maintain optimal body balance.
- **Evening Practice for Relaxation:** Dedicating time to somatic practices before going to bed can facilitate relaxation and improve sleep quality. Deep breathing exercises or muscle relaxation can help calm the mind and prepare the body for a restful night.

Continuous Awareness: Maintaining an attitude of awareness throughout the day helps recognize when the body is in a state of tension and promptly intervening with somatic exercises.

Chapter 2: Establishing a Somatic Exercise Routine

Through a series of detailed steps, this chapter will guide you in personalizing your routine, considering your specific needs, abilities, and goals. The key to an effective approach to somatic exercises lies not only in the correct execution of the exercises themselves but also in adapting and integrating the practice into the various aspects of daily life and health conditions.

2.1 Creating a Personalized Routine

Developing a personalized somatic exercise routine is crucial for maximizing the benefits of this practice. A well-structured and tailored routine can improve physical and mental health and support long-term personal growth. To create such a routine, it is essential to assess one's needs, set realistic goals, and plan an appropriate progression of exercises.

Assessing Individual Needs

The first step in creating a somatic exercise routine is accurately assessing individual needs. This process involves deep reflection on one's current health status, lifestyle habits, and any specific physical conditions. Elements to consider include:

- **Medical and Physical History**: Understanding past injuries, chronic medical conditions, or physical limitations that might affect the ability to perform certain exercises.
- **Current Fitness Level:** Evaluating one's level of flexibility, strength, and endurance to determine an appropriate starting point.
- **Specific Needs**: Identifying areas of the body that are particularly tense or weak and that could benefit most from somatic exercises.
- **Lifestyle and Availability**: Considering how many minutes or hours per week can realistically be dedicated to practice and how this fits into the daily routine.

Self-assessment should be honest and detailed, as it will provide the basis for a personalized program that effectively addresses the needs of the body and mind.

Setting Realistic Goals

Once the starting situation is understood, the next step is to set clear and realistic goals. Goals should be SMART (Specific, Measurable, Achievable, Relevant, Time-bound):

- Specific: Goals should be clear and precise. For example, instead of "improve flexibility," a more specific goal could be "increase the ability to touch toes without bending the knees."
- Measurable: It must be possible to measure progress toward the goal to maintain motivation and adjust the routine if necessary.
- Achievable: Goals must be realistic and attainable within the context of one's physical limitations and available time.
- Relevant: Goals should be meaningful for personal well-being and support broader life aspirations.
- Time-bound: Setting a deadline for achieving the goals can help maintain focus and effectively structure the routine.

Progression of Exercises

The progression of exercises in a somatic routine is essential to keep the body challenged but not overloaded. Progression should be gradual and carefully planned to avoid injuries and allow the body to adapt to new levels of physical stress:

- Gradual Start: Begin with basic exercises that require less intensity and build a fundamental body awareness.
- Gradual Increase: As the body adapts, gradually increase the intensity of the exercises, the duration of sessions, or the complexity of movements.
- Variation: Alternate exercises to stimulate different areas of the body and maintain interest. This can include introducing new somatic exercises or modifying existing ones to increase difficulty.
- Listening to the Body: Always pay attention to the body's reactions. If pain or discomfort is experienced, it is necessary to review the intensity or form of the exercise.

Creating a personalized somatic exercise routine requires a holistic approach that considers individual needs, realistic goals, and a well-planned progression of exercises. By following these steps, it is possible to develop an effective program that promotes physical and mental well-being, significantly improving quality of life.

2.2 Maintaining Motivation and Monitoring Progress

Maintaining motivation and monitoring progress are essential components for the success of any exercise program, including somatic exercises. The progressive and often subtle nature of improvements in somatic exercises can make it particularly challenging for individuals to appreciate daily changes. However, through the effective use of self-monitoring techniques, the use of technological tools like apps and workout diaries, and sharing progress with a community or coach, it is possible to not only stay motivated but also optimize the entire training experience.

Self-Monitoring Techniques

Self-monitoring is a fundamental aspect for anyone wishing to undertake a somatic exercise routine, as it allows maintaining active control over progress and adjusting practice based on the body's responses. Implementing an effective self-monitoring system requires attention to various factors that go beyond simply tracking performed exercises.

1. **Detailed Daily Log:** Keeping a daily journal is one of the most effective methods for self-monitoring. In this journal, besides recording the exercises performed, it is important to note the time dedicated to each exercise, the number of repetitions, and any modifications made to the usual routine. This helps to see not only the consistency and frequency of exercise but also how the practice evolves over time.
2. **Monitoring Physical Sensations:** Besides technical details, it is crucial to record physical sensations during and after exercises. This includes perceptions of pain, tension, relaxation, or any other significant sensation. Noting these sensations can help understand which exercises work best and which might need adjustments to avoid injuries or discomfort.
3. **Emotional Assessment**: Somatic exercises do not only affect the body but also the mind. Recording how one feels emotionally before and after exercises can offer valuable insights into the overall impact of the routine on mental health. This can include changes in mood, stress levels, and general feelings of well-being.
4. **Visual Feedback:** The use of photographs or videos can be extremely useful for visualizing progress over time. Recording oneself while performing exercises allows observing one's form and technique and noting improvements or areas that require further adjustments. This type of visual feedback is particularly useful for those working on posture and alignment.

5. **Progress Thresholds and Regression Indicators:** Defining specific progress indicators helps establish when an exercise is becoming easier or when goals are being achieved. Likewise, it is important to identify signs of possible regression or stalling, such as increased pain or decreased mobility, which could indicate the need to modify the approach.

6. **Comparison with Long-Term Goals:** Periodically, it is useful to review progress concerning established long-term goals. This helps maintain perspective on the overall path and adjust goals based on changes in lifestyle, health conditions, or simply personal preferences.

Here's a practical example:
Scenario: Alice, 40 years old, aims to improve her flexibility and reduce back pain through somatic exercises.

Specific Goals:
- Increase trunk flexibility to touch toes without bending knees.
- Reduce chronic lower back pain from moderate to mild or non-existent.

Progress Thresholds:
- **Short-term (1 month):** Alice should be able to bend and touch the middle of her shins without significant pain. This indicates improved flexibility and effective pain management.
- **Mid-term (3 months):** Alice should be able to touch her ankles while keeping her knees straight. The pain reduction should allow her to perform daily activities without discomfort.
- **Long-term (6 months):** Alice aims to touch her toes. Back pain should be rare or absent, and she should feel more agile in her daily activities.

Regression Indicators:
- **Increased Pain:** If Alice begins experiencing increased lower back pain after exercise sessions, this might indicate that exercises are too intense or performed incorrectly.
- **Decreased Mobility:** If Alice notices her ability to bend down worsens or she feels more stiffness in the morning, this could suggest the need to review and adjust the exercise routine.

Implementation and Monitoring:
- **Workout Diary:** Alice keeps a workout diary where she notes her progress, sensations during and after exercises, and perceived pain level. She uses a scale from 1 to 10 to rate the pain and notes the distance reached with her hands during forward bending.

- **Regular Evaluation Sessions:** Alice meets with her somatic therapist once a month to evaluate progress and make any necessary adjustments to her routine. During these sessions, the details of the workout diary are discussed, and a physical assessment is performed to monitor flexibility and pain.
- **Adaptation:** If Alice experiences increased pain or decreased mobility, the somatic therapist might decide to modify the difficulty of exercises by introducing slower movements or reducing the frequency of exercises involving the lower back. Additionally, complementary exercises might be introduced to strengthen abdominal muscles and improve spinal support.

Using Apps and Workout Diaries

In the digital age, apps and digital workout diaries offer powerful and convenient tools for monitoring progress. These technological resources can automate many aspects of monitoring, making it simpler and faster to record and analyze performance.

- **Fitness Apps**: Many apps allow setting specific goals, tracking exercises, time, frequency, and providing immediate feedback.
- **Digital Workout Diaries**: These diaries enable users to track their workouts, notes on sensations, thoughts during exercises, and overall progress. Many of these diaries also include analysis features that can help visualize progress over time, increasing motivation.

Using these technologies can not only facilitate data collection but also stimulate user engagement with their workout routine, making the process more interactive and rewarding.

Sharing Progress with the Community or a Coach

Another crucial aspect of maintaining motivation is sharing progress with others. This can occur in various contexts:

- **Online Communities:** Many online platforms and forums are dedicated to somatic exercises and body practices. Sharing experiences, progress, and challenges with other enthusiasts can provide support, advice, and encouragement.
- **Personal Trainers or Therapists:** Working with a professional can not only help further personalize the exercise routine but also obtain specific and qualified feedback on progress. Coaches can monitor improvements, suggest adjustments, and motivate their clients through recognition and new challenges.

Sharing progress helps create a sense of accountability and community, which are powerful motivators. Feeling part of a group or having a coach actively following one's progress can stimulate a deeper dedication to practice and transform exercise from a solitary activity into a shared and supported experience.

In conclusion, maintaining motivation and monitoring progress are essential for the long-term success of a somatic exercise routine. By using self-monitoring techniques, leveraging digital technology, and sharing the experience with others, individuals can optimize their practice, stay motivated, and achieve their health and wellness goals more effectively.

2.3 Adaptations for Different Health Conditions

Integrating somatic exercises into a training regimen may require specific adaptations to meet the needs of different health conditions, age groups, and ability levels. This subchapter offers a detailed guide on how to personalize somatic exercises to ensure both effectiveness and safety, with particular attention to the elderly, young adults, those suffering from specific conditions such as arthritis or poor posture, and general safety and precaution tips.

Advice for Seniors and Young Adults

Seniors
Seniors can greatly benefit from somatic exercises, which can significantly improve mobility, increase flexibility, and reduce pain—crucial factors for maintaining autonomy and improving quality of life at this stage. To optimize these benefits, it is essential to personalize exercises to fit individual capacities and prevent the risk of falls and other injuries.

- **Safe Supports:** Using chairs or other stable supports is essential during exercises that require balancing. These supports provide safety and allow seniors to focus on form and movement without the fear of falling, making the experience both safe and beneficial.
- **Focus on Balance and Coordination:** Integrating exercises that specifically improve balance and coordination into the daily routine is vital. Activities such as standing up from a chair without using hands or walking in a straight line can strengthen the muscles involved in balance, reducing the risk of falls, which are a major cause of serious injuries among seniors.
- **Gentle and Fluid Movements:** It is important to include exercises that promote wide and fluid joint movements, such as gentle stretching and slow rotations, which can help maintain or even improve joint mobility without putting excessive stress on the joints. These movements also help lubricate the joints and keep connective tissue flexible.

Young Adults

Young adults may face challenges related to a sedentary lifestyle or stress from work and study. Somatic exercises offer an effective solution for managing stress and preventing musculoskeletal problems that can arise from prolonged and inadequate postures.

- **Counteracting Sedentary Lifestyle:** It is beneficial to incorporate short and manageable somatic exercises during work or study breaks. Light stretching exercises, fluid movements, or deep breathing exercises can be performed in a few minutes but provide significant refreshment and help keep the body active and the mind clear.
- **Relaxation Routine:** Promoting a routine that includes exercises specifically for muscle relaxation and tension reduction is essential. Techniques such as diaphragmatic breathing or guided meditation can be particularly effective in neutralizing the effects of psychological stress and improving overall emotional well-being.
- **Habit Promotion:** It is crucial to develop a regular routine of somatic exercises that not only helps combat sedentary lifestyle but also serves as a foundation for an active and healthy lifestyle. Encouraging the integration of these exercises into daily life can help young adults establish healthy habits that will endure over time, reducing the risk of long-term health problems associated with an inactive and stressful lifestyle.

Modifications for Those with Specific Conditions

Arthritis: Individuals with arthritis can greatly benefit from somatic exercises, which help reduce joint stiffness and pain. Recommended adaptations include:

- Avoiding movements that place excessive stress on inflamed joints.
- Including exercises that promote smooth movements and stretching, keeping the joints mobile without overloading them.
- Using breathing and mental awareness exercises to help manage pain and anxiety associated with the condition.

Poor Posture: For those suffering from poor posture, often due to bad daily habits, somatic exercises can help realign and strengthen the body:

- Focus on exercises that strengthen the core and improve spinal alignment.
- Implement routines that specifically target problem areas, such as the upper back and shoulders, to correct imbalances.
- Educate on the importance of correct posture through increased body awareness during exercises.

Safety Precautions and Tips

Regardless of health condition, age, or fitness level, it is essential to adopt precautions to ensure that somatic exercises are practiced safely:

- **Medical Consultation:** Before starting any new exercise program, especially in the presence of pre-existing medical conditions, it is important to consult a healthcare professional to obtain approval.
- **Listening to the Body:** It is crucial to pay attention to the body's signals and stop if pain or discomfort is felt. Somatic exercises are designed to be gentle and should never cause pain.
- **Safe Environment:** Ensure that the practice area is free of obstacles and hazards, with a stable surface and adequate support equipment if necessary.
- **Gradual Increase:** Gradually increase the duration and intensity of exercises to avoid overload and injuries.
- **Professional Guidance:** Consider working with a qualified somatic exercise instructor, especially in the initial stages, to ensure movements are performed correctly and safely.

Part II: Practical Exercises

Chapter 3: Anti-Stress Exercises

3.1 Exercises for Body Awareness (Grounding)

Seated Body Scan (No.1)

Objective: Improve interoceptive awareness and relax the body by focusing attention on each part while seated.

Scan this QRcode to direct access on exercise!

STEP 1: Sit straight on a chair, close your eyes, and focus on your breath.

STEP 2: Mentally scan your body, noting any tension and movement with your breath.

STEP 3: Stay in position for a few seconds.

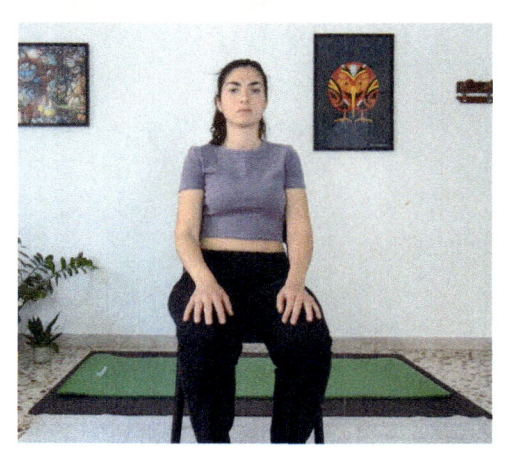

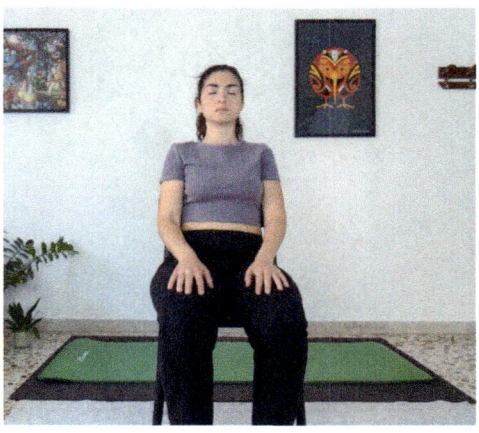

Breath Exploration (No. 2)

Objective: Increase the ability to control and use the breath effectively.

STEP 1: Lie on a mat with arms and legs relaxed, and observe your breath.

STEP 2: Focus on the movement of the chest and abdomen, feeling the air come in and out.

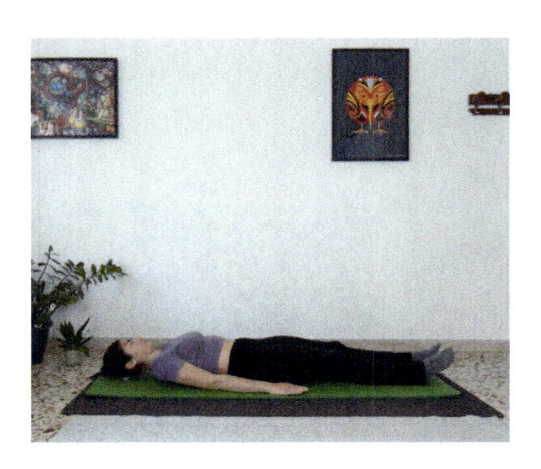

STEP 3: Stay in position for a few seconds.

Standing Posture Alignment (No. 3)

Objective: Develop awareness of your posture while standing to improve balance and reduce muscle tension.

Scan this QRcode to direct access on exercise!

STEP 1: Stand with feet shoulder-width apart and back straight for a few seconds.

STEP 2: Ensure your head is aligned with your spine and shoulders are relaxed.

STEP 3: Notice the weight distribution on your feet and maintain an even balance.

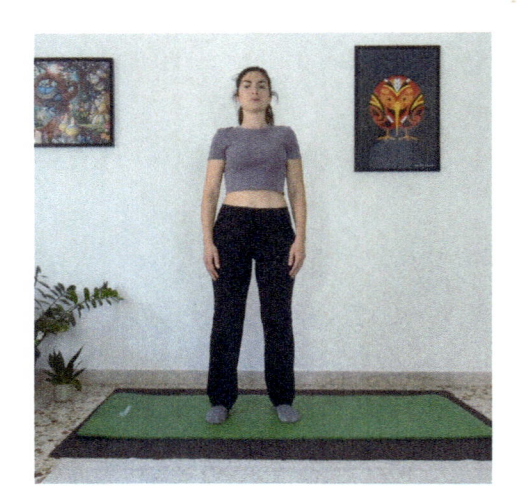

Awareness of Hands and Arms (No. 4)

Objective: Increase sensitivity and control of hand and arm movements to improve coordination.

STEP 1: Sit or stand, focusing on your hands and arms.

STEP 2: Slowly move your hands and fingers, noting any tension or relaxation.

STEP 3: Observe the movement of your arms in space and their responsiveness to mental commands.

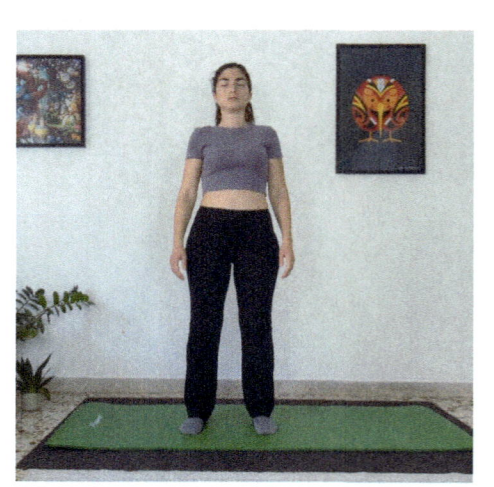

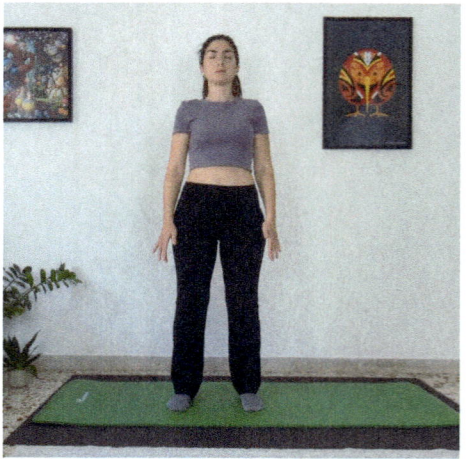

Exploring Spine Flexibility (No. 5)

Objective: *Improve spinal mobility to increase fluidity and reduce the risk of injuries.*

STEP 1: Lie on your back with knees bent and feet on the floor.

STEP 2: Focus on your spine and slowly rotate your pelvis and lower back from side to side, exploring the flexibility of your spine.

STEP 3: Repeat for 15 seconds.

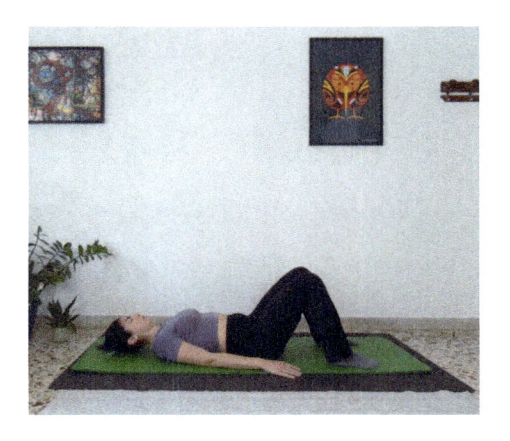

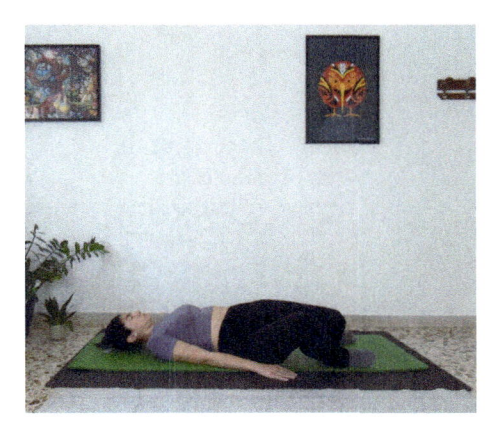

Scan this QRcode to direct access on exercise!

Awareness of Feet and Ankles (No. 6)

Objective: *Increase perception and stability of the feet and ankles, improving the support base for the entire body.*

STEP 1: Sit or stand.

STEP 2: Raise and lower your toes, feeling the movement in your ankles.

STEP 3: Notice the contact of your feet with the floor and how they respond to movements.

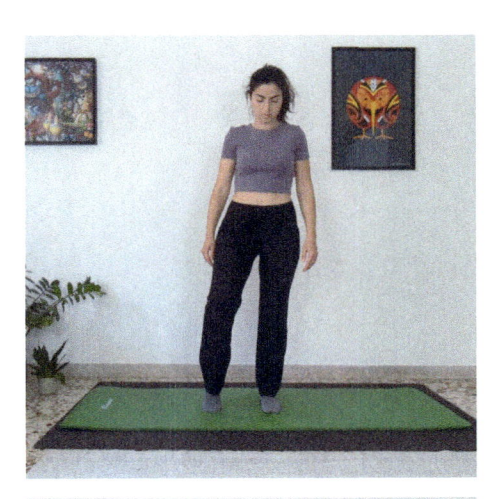

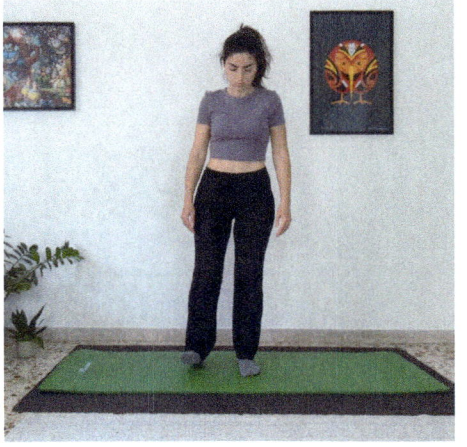

3.2 Exercises for Muscle Relaxation

Neck and Shoulders

Neck Extension Stretch (No. 7)

Objective: Relieve tension in the back of the neck and improve neck flexibility.

STEP 1: Sit or stand with your back straight.

STEP 2: Gently tilt your head back, looking up.

STEP 3: Hold for 15 seconds, then slowly return to a neutral position.

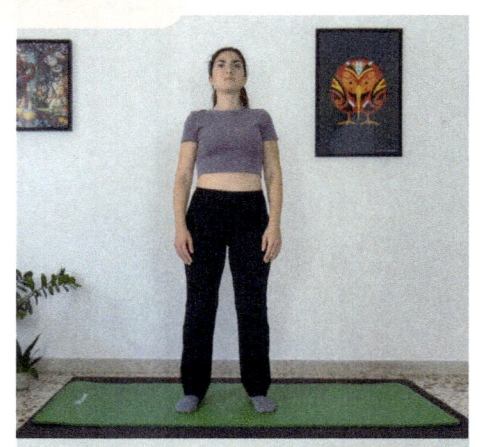

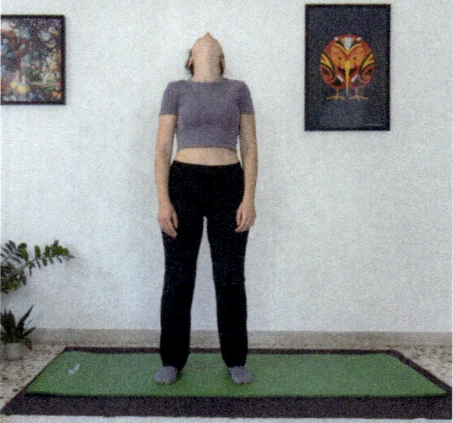

Scan this QRcode to direct access on exercise!

Neck Rotation (No. 8)

Objective: Improve neck mobility and flexibility, reducing tension and increasing the range of motion through controlled rotations.

STEP 1: Sit or stand.

STEP 2: Slowly rotate your neck from side to side, keeping your shoulders relaxed and your chin parallel to the floor.

STEP 3: Repeat 5 times on each side.

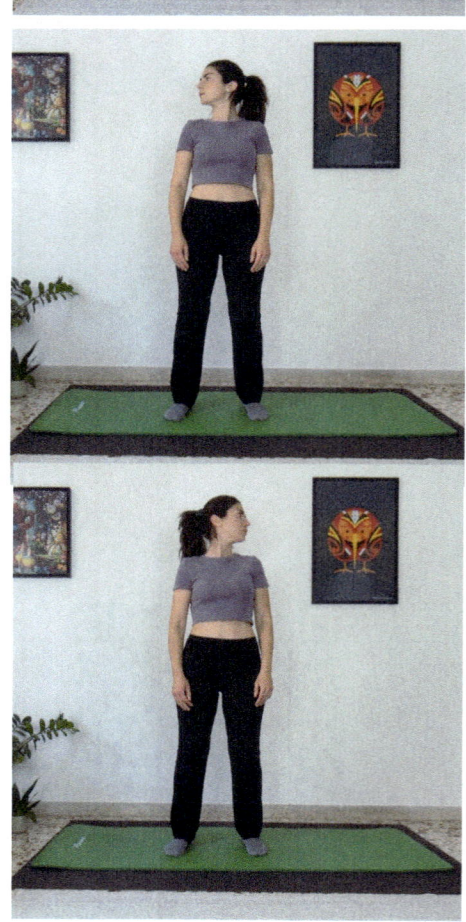

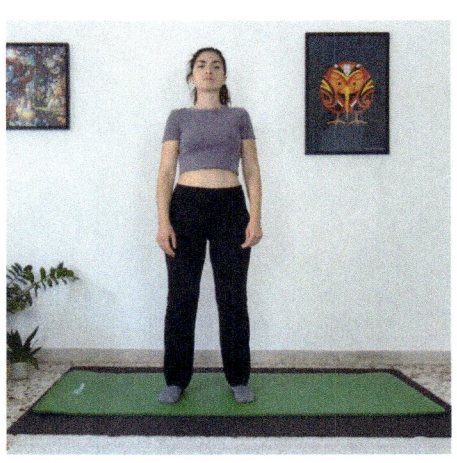

Neck and Shoulders

Chin to Chest Stretch (No. 9)

Objective: Relax the neck and upper back muscles.

Scan this QRcode to direct access on exercise!

STEP 1: Sit or stand with your back straight.

STEP 2: Slowly lower your chin towards your chest until you feel a stretch in the back of your neck.

STEP 3: Hold for 10 seconds and release. Repeat 5 times.

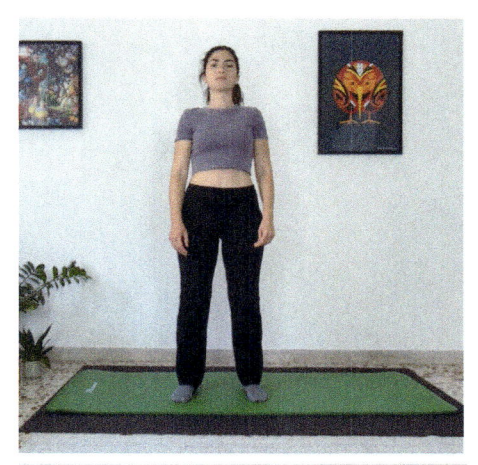

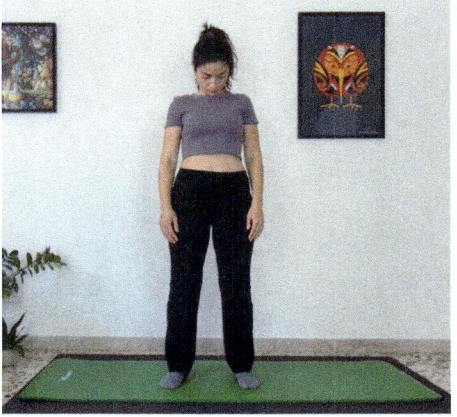

Shoulder Lifts (No. 10)

Objective: Strengthen and relax the shoulder muscles through repeated lifts, helping to release accumulated stress and tension.

STEP 1: Sit or stand.

STEP 2: Inhale as you slowly lift your shoulders towards your ears, holding the tension for a few seconds.

STEP 3: Exhale and release your shoulders down.

STEP 4: Repeat 8 times.

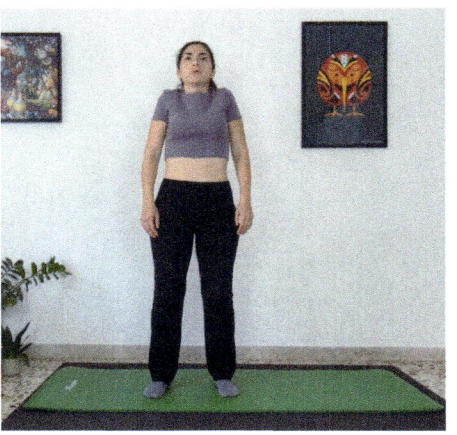

Neck and Shoulders

Shoulder Rotation (No. 11)

Objective: Increase circulation and flexibility of the shoulders with circular movements, improving shoulder joint mobility.

STEP 1: Stand with arms at your sides.

STEP 2: Slowly rotate your shoulders forward in a circular motion a few times.

STEP 3: Then rotate them backward.

STEP 4: Repeat 10-12 times in both directions.

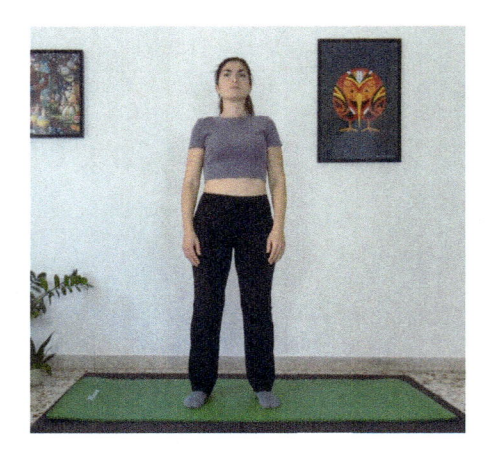

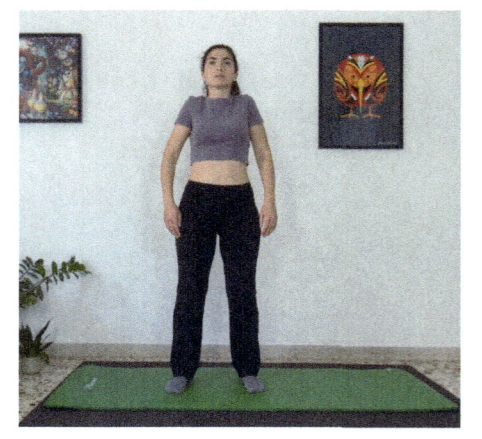

Scan this QRcode to direct access on exercise!

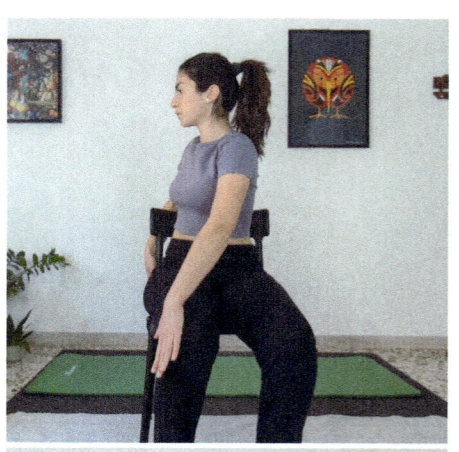

Back and Lower Back Pain

Seated Thoracic Rotation (No. 12)

Objective: Increase thoracic spine mobility and improve trunk flexibility through controlled rotations while seated.

STEP 1: Sit on a chair with both feet on the ground.

STEP 2: Place one hand on the left side of the chair near your hip and slowly rotate your torso to the left, bringing the other hand (right) to your left knee.

STEP 3: Hold for a few seconds and breathe deeply.

STEP 4: Repeat 5 times on each side.

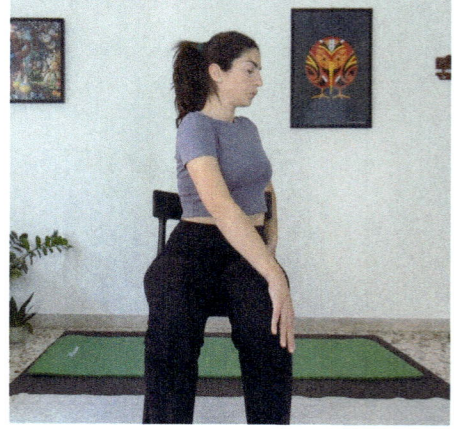

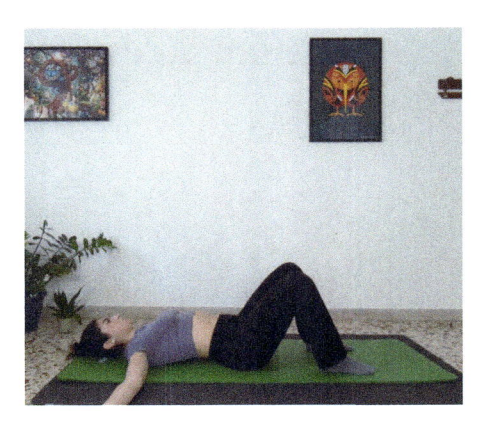

Back and Lower Back Pain

Child's Pose (No. 13)

Objective: Relax the back and lower back, relieving tension and stress.

STEP 1: Start on your knees with your buttocks on your heels.

STEP 2: Extend your arms forward and lower your torso between your thighs, resting your forehead on the ground.

STEP 3: Hold for 20 seconds and return to the starting position.

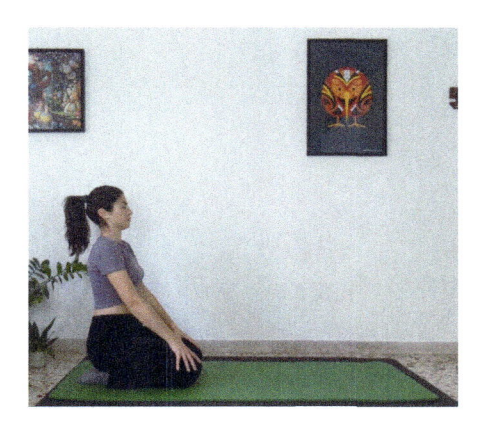

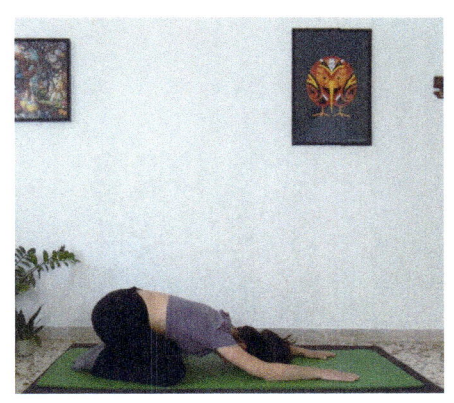

Scan this QRcode to direct access on exercise!

Lower Back Twist (No. 14)

Objective: Relieve lower back tension and improve spinal mobility.

STEP 1: Lie on your back with knees bent and feet flat on the floor.

STEP 2: Extend your arms to form a T and rotate both knees to one side, keeping your shoulders on the ground.

STEP 3: Hold for 20 seconds, then switch sides.

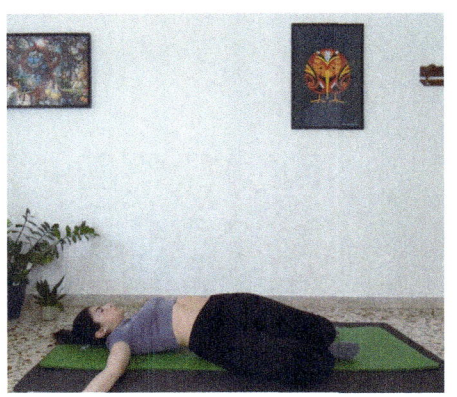

Back and Lower Back Pain

Seated Neck Stretch (No. 15)

Objective: Relieve neck tension and improve the range of motion.

Scan this QRcode to direct access on exercise!

STEP 1: Sit straight on a chair, feet on the ground, shoulders relaxed.

STEP 2: Slowly turn your neck to the right, hold for 3 seconds; return to the center and repeat to the left.

STEP 3: Lower your chin to your chest, hold for 3 seconds; raise your chin, hold for 3 seconds.

STEP 4: Repeat 5 times.

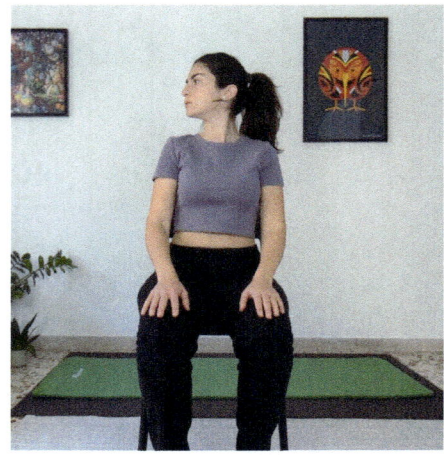

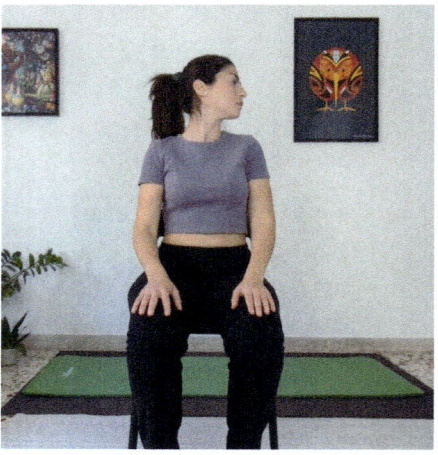

Glute Stretch (No. 16)

Objective: Improve glute muscle flexibility and relieve tension and pain in the lower back and hips.

STEP 1: Lie on your back with knees bent.

STEP 2: Place your right foot on your left thigh and grab behind your left thigh.

STEP 3: Pull your left leg towards you, feeling the stretch in your right glute, and hold for 20 seconds.

STEP 4: Switch sides and repeat 2 times per side.

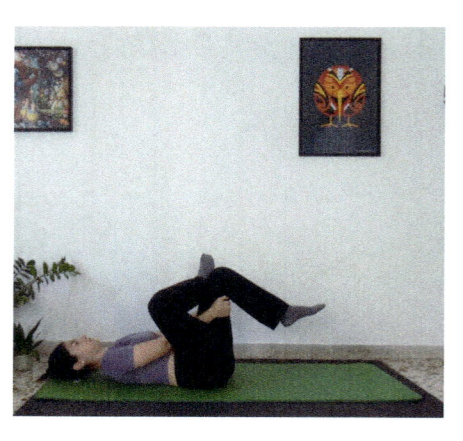

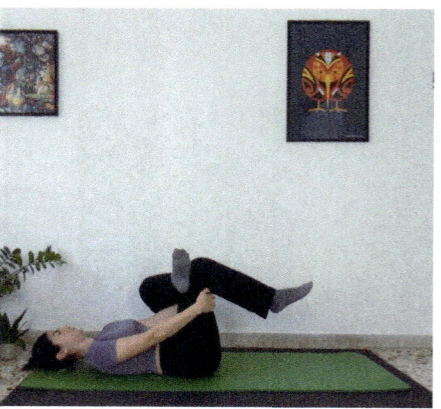

Lower and Upper Limbs

Calf Stretch (No. 17)

Objective: Improve elasticity and reduce tension in calf muscles, promoting better ankle mobility and preventing injuries related to running and other physical activities.

STEP 1: Stand facing a wall or on a stable support.
STEP 2: Place one foot back and slightly bend your knee.

STEP 3: Rest your hands on the wall and push the heel to the ground, feeling the stretch in your back calf.

STEP 4: Hold for 20 seconds, then switch sides. Repeat 5 times per side.

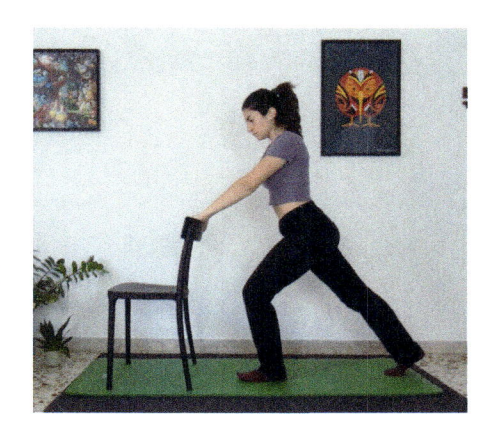

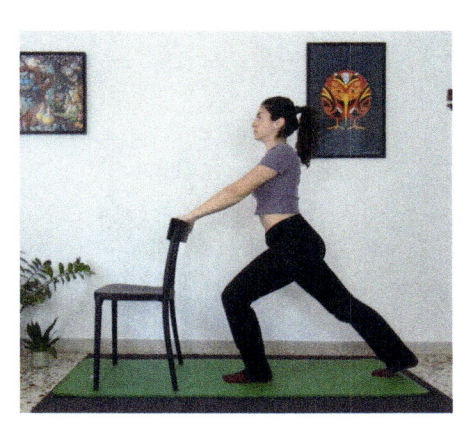

Scan this QRcode to direct access on exercise!

Seated Leg Cross Stretch (No. 18)

Objective: Relax the muscles of the lower back and hip.

STEP 1: Sit on a chair, keeping your back straight.

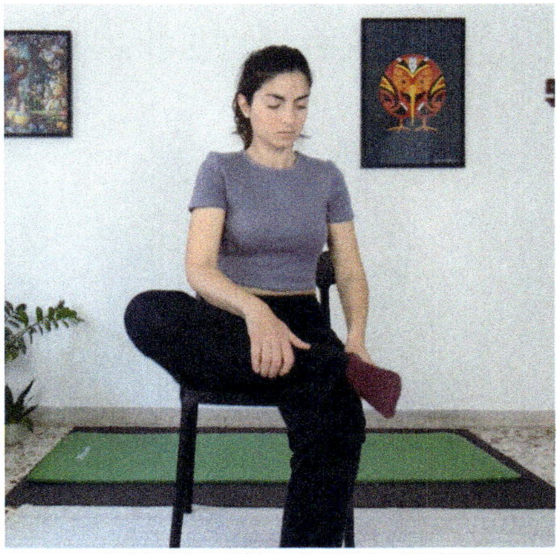

STEP 2: Place one ankle on the opposite thigh, forming a 90-degree angle with the crossed leg.

STEP 3: Apply gentle pressure on the crossed thigh with your hand and lean forward to intensify the stretch.

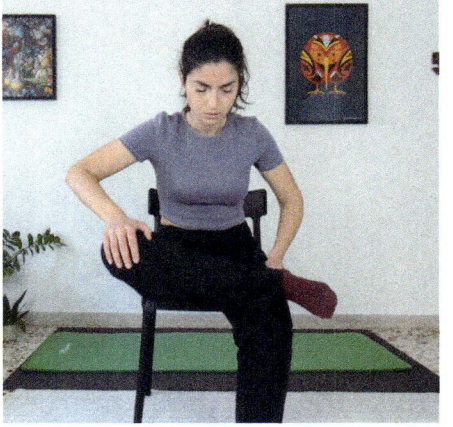

Lower and Upper Limbs

Upper Back and Shoulder Stretch (No. 19)

Objective: Relax and stretch the muscles of the upper back and shoulders.

Scan this QRcode to direct access on exercise!

STEP 1: Stand or sit with your back straight.

STEP 2: Interlace your hands and extend them in front of you, palm to palm, with arms parallel to the floor.

STEP 3: Push your hands forward while rounding your back, pushing your spine towards the wall behind you, and lower your head between your arms.
Hold for 15 seconds. Repeat 5 times.

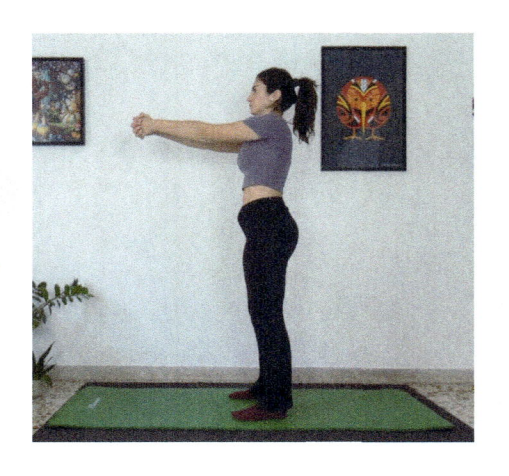

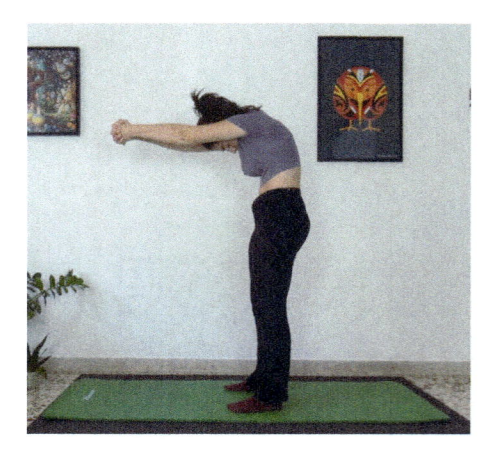

Pectoral Stretch (No. 20)

Objective: Increase flexibility of the chest muscles and help correct body posture by reducing tension in the pectoral muscles, often shortened by prolonged computer use or poor posture.

STEP 1: Stand with your arms behind your back.

STEP 2: Interlace your hands and lift your arms slightly upwards, feeling the stretch in your chest and shoulders.

STEP 3: Hold for 20 seconds, then release. Repeat 5 times.

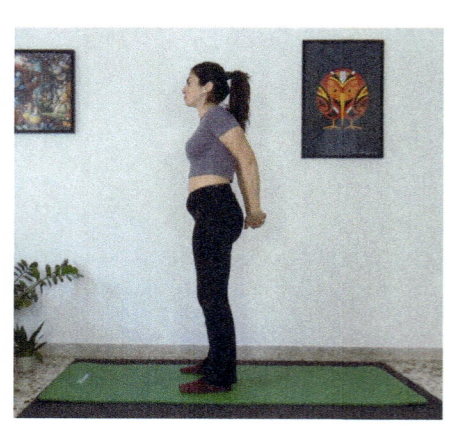

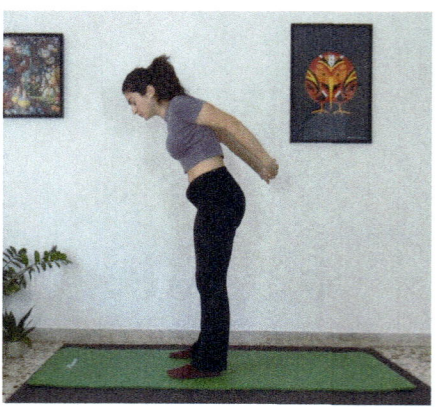

3.3 Exercises for Chronic Pain

When suffering from **chronic pain**, physical exercise can seem like a daunting challenge. However, specific and controlled movements can help manage pain, improve mobility, and strengthen muscles safely. It is important to **start gradually**, always listening to your body, and avoiding movements that cause acute pain. A slow and steady approach is crucial to ensuring that physical activity is beneficial and not aggravating. Always consult a healthcare professional before starting any exercise program.

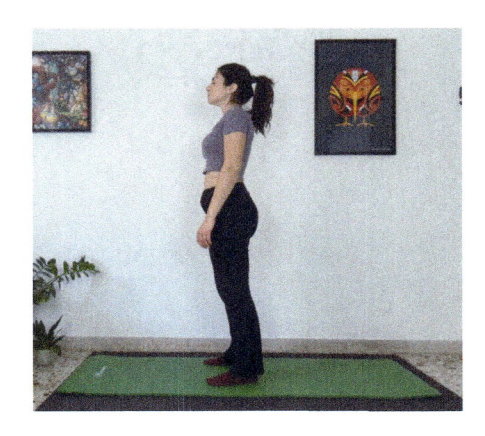

Neck and Shoulders

Chin Tucks (No. 21)

Objective: Reduce neck tension, improve posture, and alleviate shoulder pain.

Scan this QRcode to direct access on exercise!

STEP 1: Sit or stand with your back straight.

STEP 2: Pull your chin back towards your neck as if making a double chin.

STEP 3: Hold for 5 seconds and then relax. Repeat 5 times.

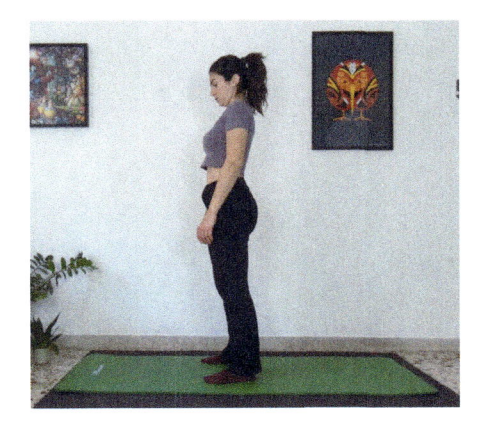

Neck and Shoulders

Arm Wall Stretch (No. 22)

Objective: Relieve tension in the shoulders and upper back.

STEP 1: Stand facing a wall and place your hands on the wall above your head.

STEP 2: Slowly bend your torso forward, keeping your hands on the wall, feeling the stretch in your shoulders, and return to the starting position. Repeat 5 times.

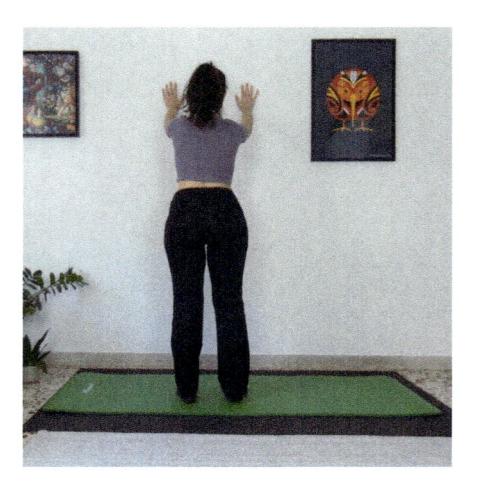

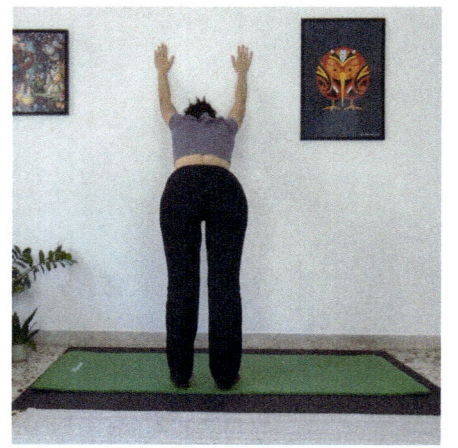

Scan this QRcode to direct access on exercise!

Back and Lower Back Pain

Seated Lower Back Stretch (No. 23)

Objective: Reduce lower back pain and improve flexibility.

STEP 1: Sit on a chair with your feet flat on the ground.

STEP 2: Lean your torso forward and reach your feet with your hands.

STEP 3: Hold for 20 seconds and slowly release. Repeat 5 times.

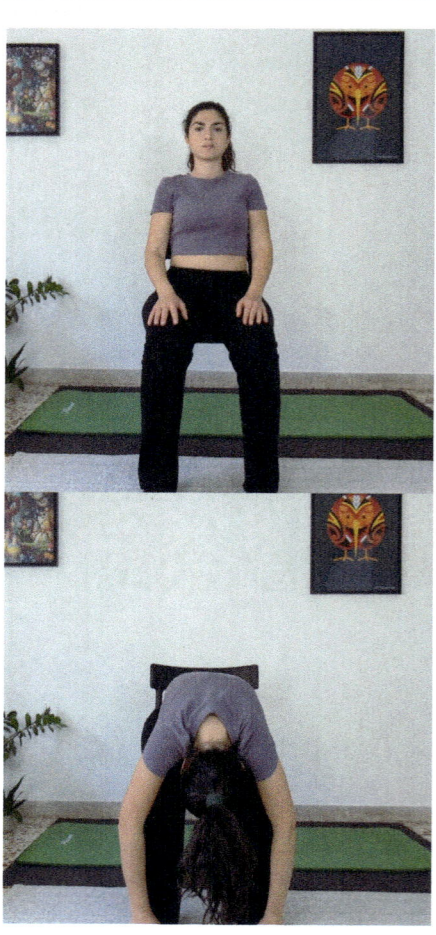

Neck and Shoulders

Pelvic Lift (No. 24)

***Objective**: Relieve lower back pain by strengthening lumbar muscles.*

Scan this QRcode to direct access on exercise!

STEP 1: Lie on your back with knees bent and feet on the ground.

STEP 2: Lift your hips towards the ceiling, forming a straight line from shoulders to knees.

STEP 3: Hold for 5 seconds, then lower slowly. Repeat 5 times.

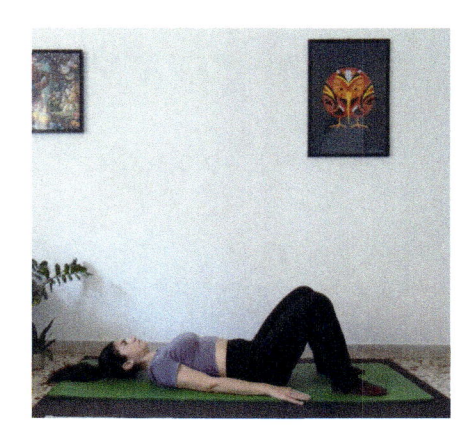

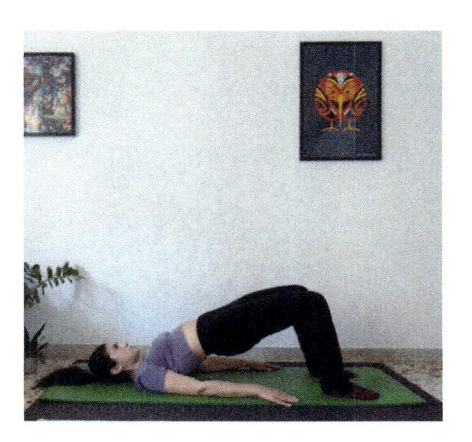

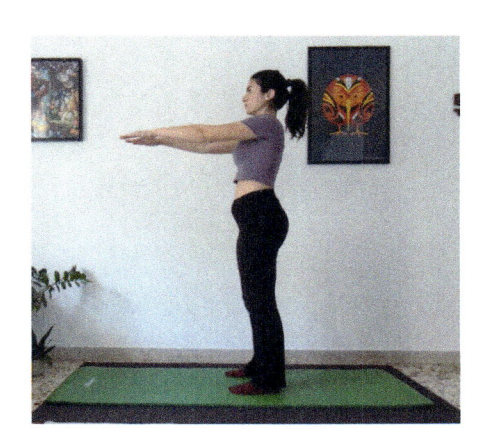

Lower and Upper Limbs

Heel Slides (No. 25)

***Objective:** Relieve tension in leg muscles and improve mobility of legs and ankles.*

STEP 1: Lie on your back on a mat with knees bent and feet flat on the floor.

STEP 2: Slowly slide one heel along the mat, extending the leg straight in front of you.

STEP 3: Slide the heel back to the starting position and repeat with the other leg 5 times per side.

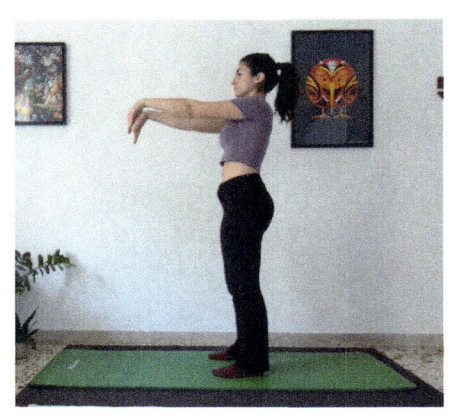

Lower and Upper Limbs

Gentle Wrist Flexion/Extension (No. 26)

Objective: *Reduce pain and improve wrist flexibility.*

Scan this QRcode to direct access on exercise!

STEP 1: Sit or stand with your arm extended and hand in a neutral position.

STEP 2: Slowly flex your wrist downward, then extend it upward for 10 repetitions.

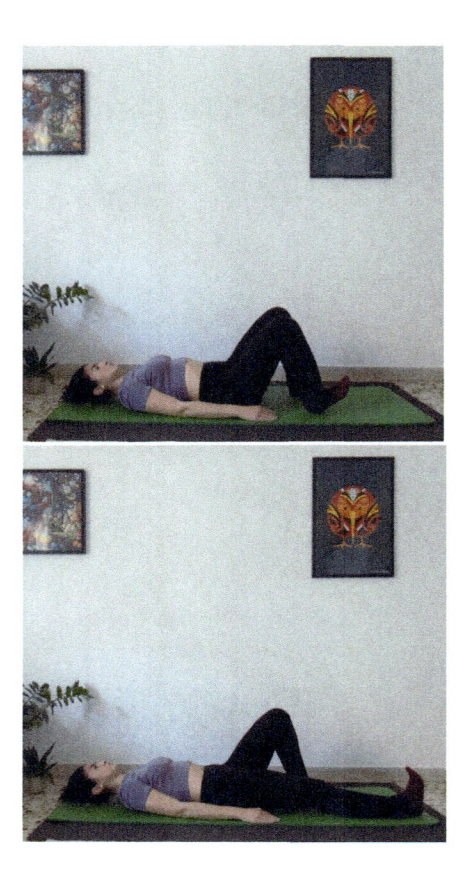

3.4 Exercises to Improve Mobility and Flexibility

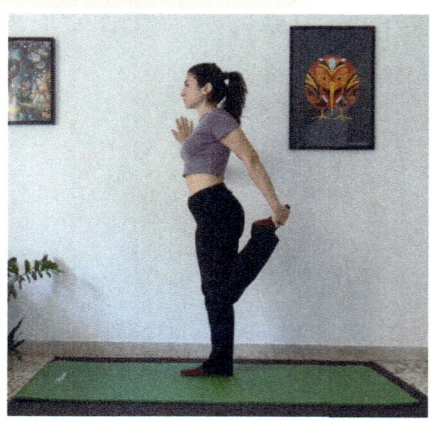

Dynamic Stretching

Standing Quad Stretch (No. 27)

Objective: *Improve quadriceps flexibility, relieve tension in the front of the thigh, and prevent injuries related to physical activity.*

STEP 1: Stand, hold onto a support with one hand, and with the other, grab the ankle of one leg and bring the heel towards the buttock, keeping your torso upright.

STEP 2: Hold for a few seconds.

STEP 3: Switch legs and repeat 8 times per side.

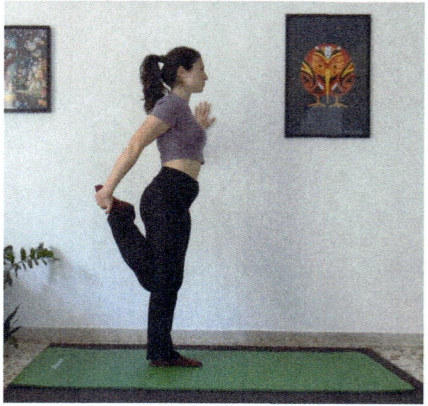

Dynamic Stretching

Knee to Chest (No. 28)

Objective: *Increase hip mobility and stretch lower back muscles, helping reduce lower back pain and improve posture.*

Scan this QRcode to direct access on exercise!

STEP 1: Stand and lift one leg bent towards your chest.

STEP 2: Hold for a few seconds and lower the leg.

STEP 3: Repeat with the other leg 5 times.

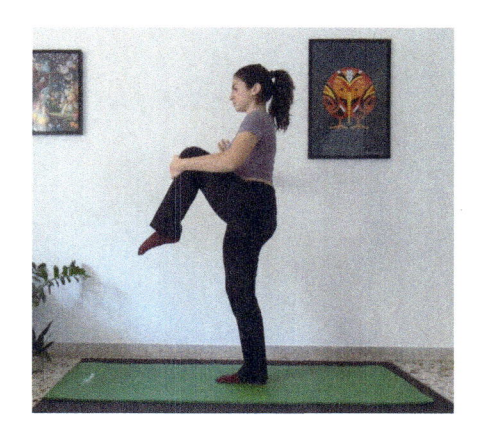

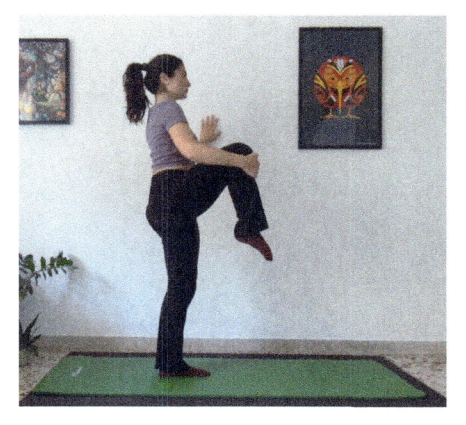

Dynamic Stretching

Arm Cross Swings (No. 29)

Objective: *Increase blood circulation and shoulder mobility.*

STEP 1: Stand with legs shoulder-width apart and bring your arms forward, crossing your wrists.

STEP 2: Swing your arms back and forth, alternating right arm over left and vice versa.

STEP 3: Do 10 swings per side.

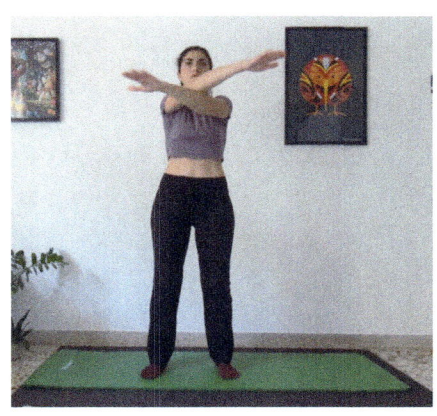

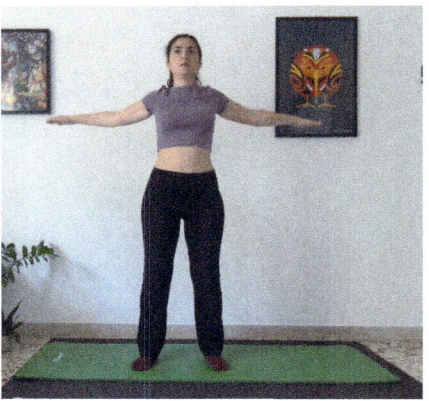

Dynamic Stretching

Lunges with Torso Twist (No. 30)

Objective: Improve leg strength, hip and spinal mobility, and overall coordination.

STEP 1: Stand, step forward with a long step, bending the front knee and keeping the back heel lifted.

STEP 2: Twist your torso towards the side of the front leg.

STEP 3: Return to the starting position and perform 10 repetitions per side.

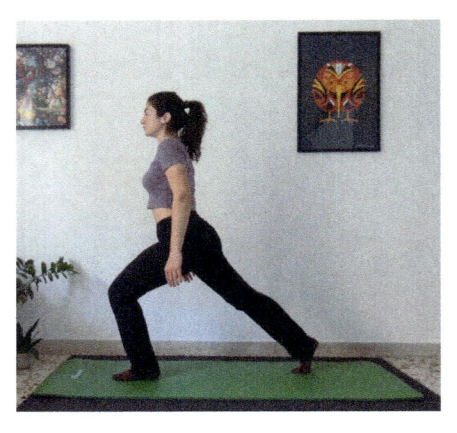

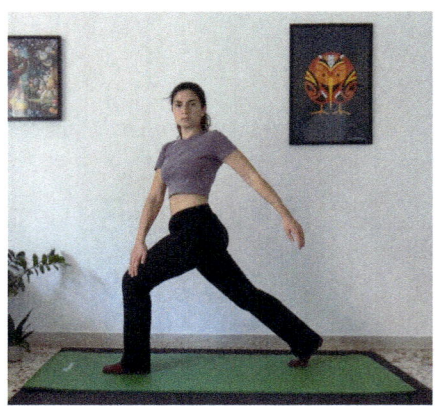

Scan this QRcode to direct access on exercise!

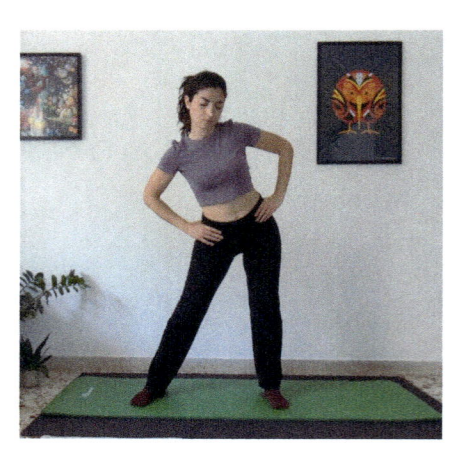

Fluid Joint Movements

Circle Hips (No. 31)

Objective: Improve hip mobility, relieve lower back tension, and increase circulation in the pelvic area.

STEP 1: Stand with feet shoulder-width apart.

STEP 2: Rotate your hips in wide circles clockwise and then counterclockwise.

STEP 3: Do 10 circles in each direction.

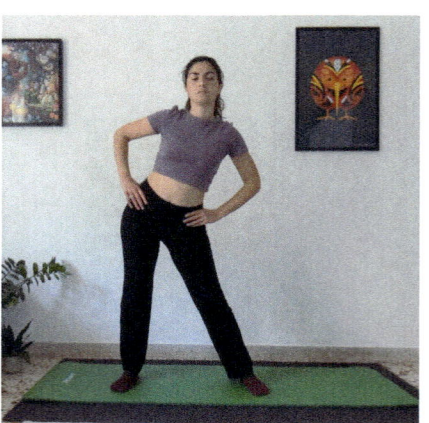

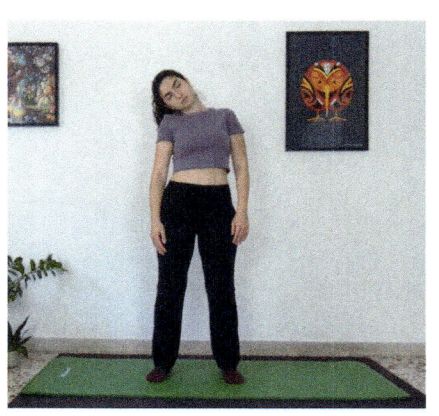

Fluid Joint Movements

Calf Raises (No. 32)

Objective: Improve ankle mobility and strengthen calves, contributing to better stability and support during walking or other physical activities.

STEP 1: Stand with feet shoulder-width apart, hold onto support if needed.

STEP 2: Slowly lift your heels until standing on your toes, maintaining the maximum extension for a few seconds.

STEP 3: Lower your heels back to the floor.

Beginner: 10 raises x 2 sets.
Intermediate: 15 x 2 sets.
Advanced: 15 x 3 sets.

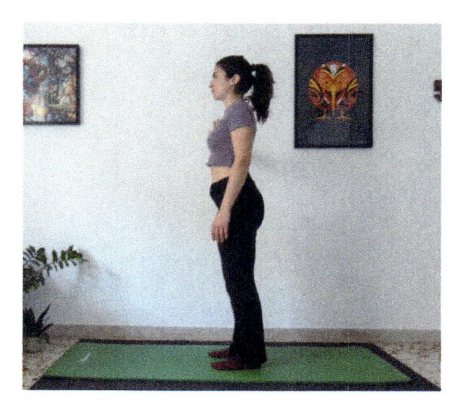

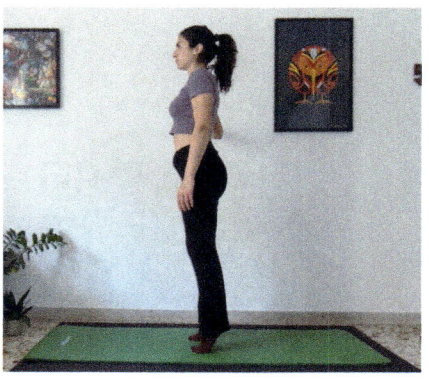

Scan this QRcode to direct access on exercise!

Neck Rolls (No. 33)

Objective: Reduce stiffness and muscle tension, increasing blood circulation and neck flexibility.

STEP 1: Stand or sit with your back straight, slowly tilt your head to one side.

STEP 2: Roll your chin across your chest to the other side.

STEP 3: Perform 5 rolls per side.

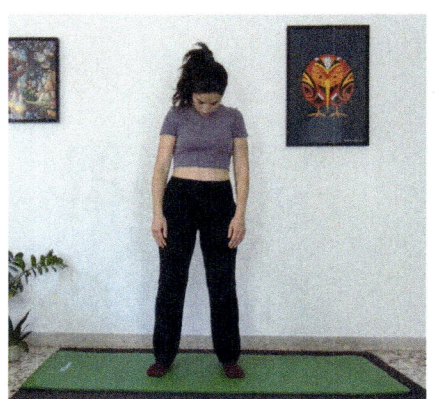

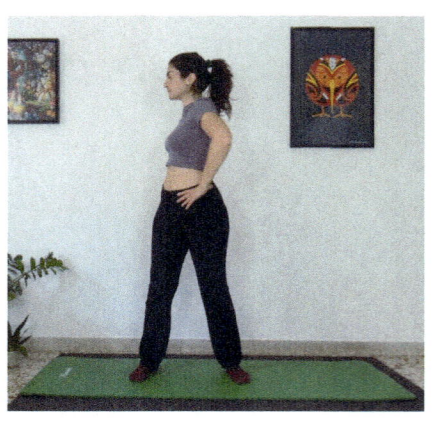

Fluid Joint Movements

Wrist Circles (No. 34)

Objective: Prevent issues like carpal tunnel by improving wrist mobility and flexibility, especially for those who work a lot on the computer.

Scan this QRcode to direct access on exercise!

STEP 1: Stand, extend your arms in front of you with palms facing down.

STEP 2: Rotate your wrists in wide circles clockwise and counterclockwise.

STEP 3: Do 10 circles in each direction.

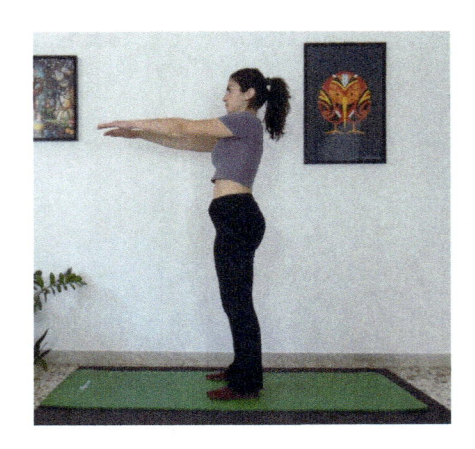

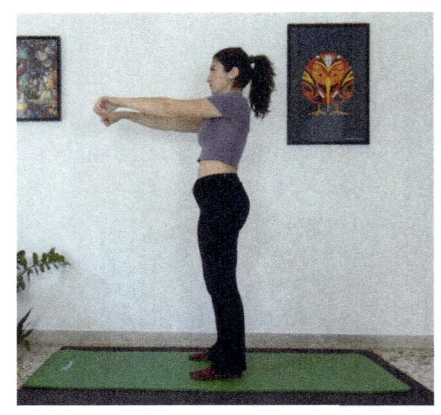

Torso Twists (No. 35)

Objective: Improve spinal mobility, strengthen abdominal and lower back muscles, and improve digestion by stimulating internal organs.

STEP 1: Stand with feet shoulder-width apart and hands on your hips.

STEP 2: Twist your torso from side to side, keeping your feet stationary.

STEP 3: Do 10 twists per side.

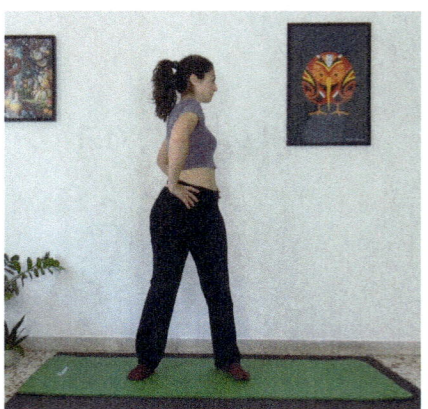

Fluid Joint Movements

Toe Taps (No. 36)

Objective: Improve circulation in the legs, increase foot and ankle flexibility, and strengthen leg muscles.

STEP 1: Sit on a chair, lift one foot off the floor.

STEP 2: Tap the floor with your toes and then lift them up.

STEP 3: Repeat 10 times per side.

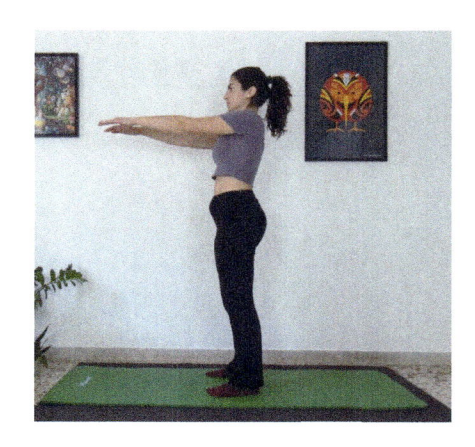

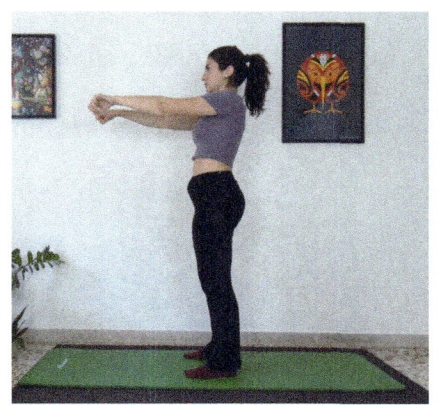

Scan this QRcode to direct access on exercise!

3.5 Pre-Sleep Exercises

Deep Breathing (No. 37)

Objective: Reduce stress and calm the mind, preparing the body for restorative sleep.

STEP 1: Lie down on your bed and place your hands on your abdomen.

STEP 2: Close your eyes and inhale slowly, counting to four.

STEP 3: Hold your breath for four seconds, then exhale slowly, counting to eight.

Repeat: Continue for 5-10 minutes.

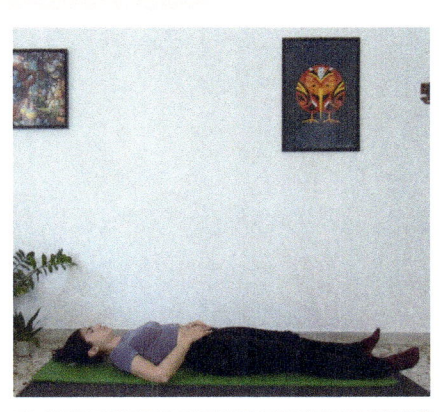

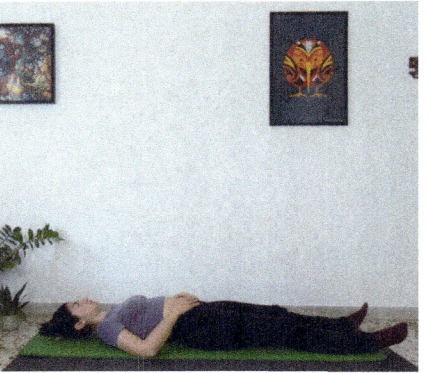

Abdominal Self-Massage (No. 38)

Objective: Reduce abdominal tension, improving pre-sleep digestion.

Scan this QRcode to direct access on exercise!

STEP 1: Lie down on your bed and place your hands on your abdomen.

STEP 2: Close your eyes and inhale slowly.

STEP 3: As you feel your abdomen rise, massage your abdomen with one hand in a circular motion.

Repeat: Continue for 5 minutes.

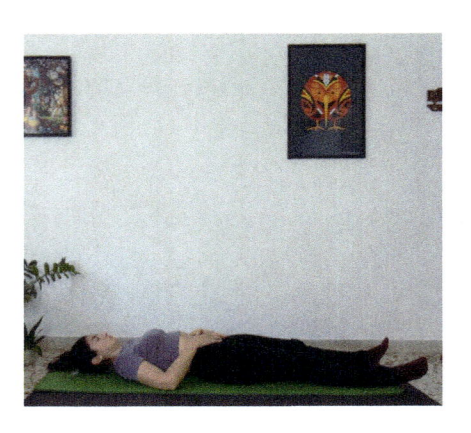

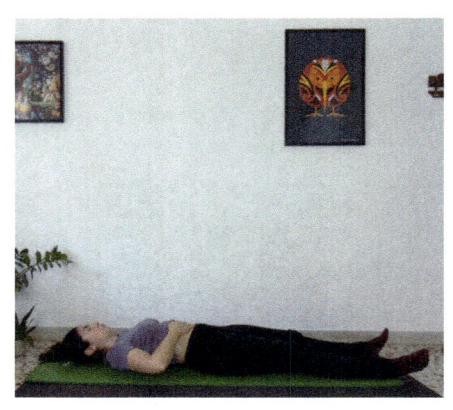

Gentle Leg Stretches (No. 39)

Objective: Reduce leg tension and promote relaxation before sleeping.

STEP 1: Lie on your back with your legs extended.

STEP 2: Slowly lift one leg, keeping it straight, and gently pull it towards you with your hands under your knee.

STEP 3: Hold the position for a few seconds and repeat with the other leg. Repeat 2 times for each leg.

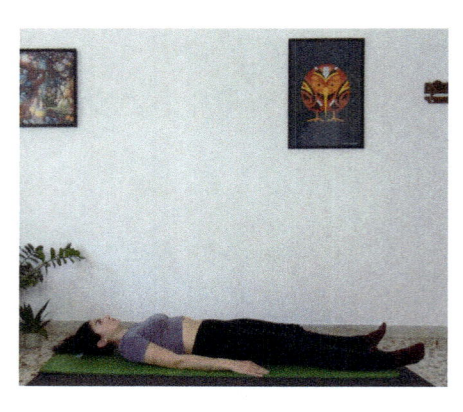

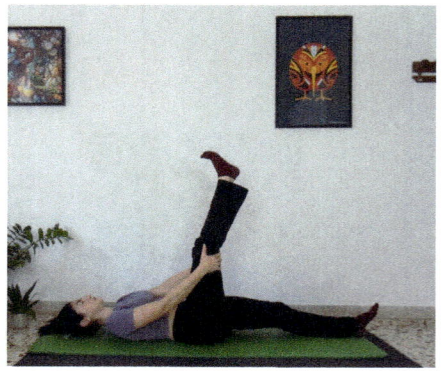

Pillow Between Legs Squeeze (No. 40)

Objective: Reduce lower back tension and align the hips during sleep, helping to relax the adductor muscles and pelvic region.

Scan this QRcode to direct access on exercise!

STEP 1: Lie on your back with your knees bent and a pillow positioned between your knees.

STEP 2: Gently squeeze the pillow between your knees, activating the inner thigh muscles without creating tension.

STEP 3: Maintain the gentle squeeze for 10 seconds, then release.

Repeat: 5-6 times.

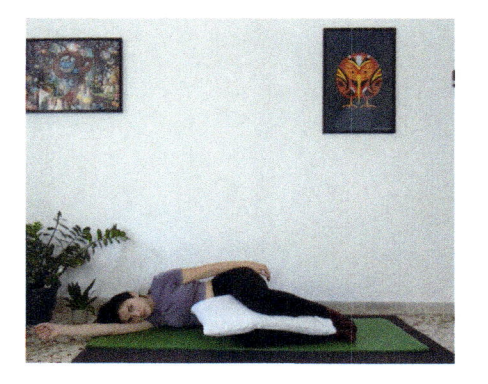

Pillow Chest Hug (No. 41)

Objective: Relax the chest and shoulder muscles, promoting a sense of comfort and security that facilitates pre-sleep relaxation.

STEP 1: Lie on your back, hugging a pillow to your chest with both arms.

STEP 2: Breathe deeply, feeling your chest expand against the pillow with each inhale.

STEP 3: Maintain the hug and deep breathing for 2-3 minutes.

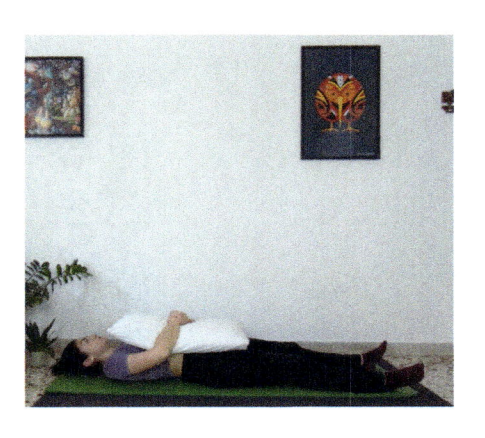

Bedtime Spinal Twist (No. 42)

Objective: Relieve tension in the spine and improve digestion.

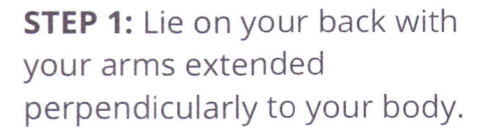

STEP 1: Lie on your back with your arms extended perpendicularly to your body.

STEP 2: Bring your knees to your chest, then let them gently fall to one side, keeping your shoulders in contact with the bed.

STEP 3: Hold the twist for 20 seconds, then switch sides.

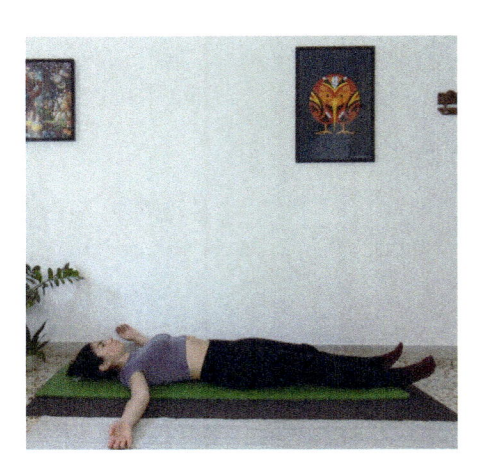

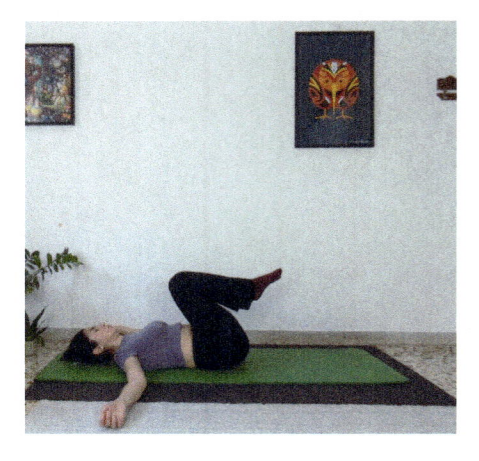

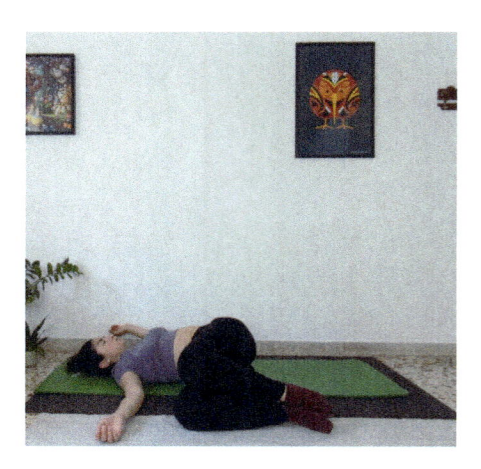

Scan this QRcode to direct access on exercise!

Chapter 4: Warming Up

Warming up exercises before a workout perform several crucial functions to prepare the body for the intense physical activity to follow.

- Increase body temperature: Warming up gradually increases body temperature, which is essential for optimizing muscle performance. A warmer body promotes smoother joint movements, reduces the risk of injury, and improves muscle efficiency.
- Improve blood circulation: During warming up, blood flow to the muscles increases, providing them with more oxygen and essential nutrients for proper functioning. This helps prepare the muscles for the effort that will follow during the main workout.
- Activate the nervous system: Warming up exercises also prepare the nervous system for the upcoming physical activity, enhancing communication between the brain and muscles. This helps improve coordination, responsiveness, and control of movement during the workout.
- Reduce the risk of injury: A proper warm-up significantly reduces the risk of muscle, tendon, and joint injuries during exercise. Warming up muscles increases their elasticity and flexibility, reducing the likelihood of strains or sprains.
- Mentally prepare the athlete: Warming up exercises not only prepare the body physically but also mentally. They help athletes focus on the upcoming workout, concentrate on bodily sensations, and mentally prepare for the physical effort to follow.

4.1 Mobility and Flexibility Exercises Pre-Workout

Side Bends (No. 43)

Objective: Increase the flexibility and mobility of the lateral spine, improve circulation, and reduce stiffness in the hips and intercostal muscles.

STEP 1: Stand with feet shoulder-width apart, back straight, arms at your sides.

STEP 2: Bend your torso laterally, sliding your hand down the corresponding leg.

STEP 3: Return to the upright position and repeat 3 times on each side.

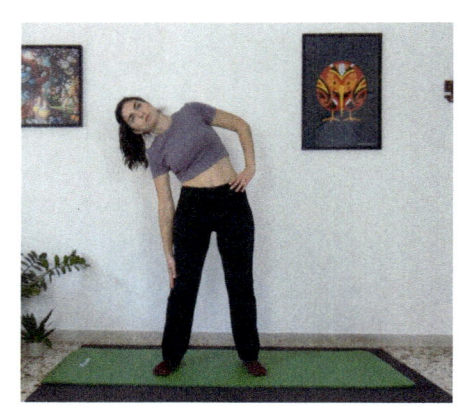

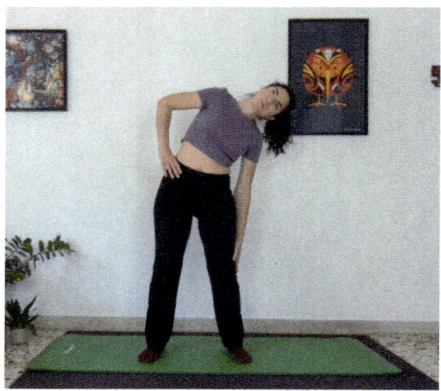

Scan this QRcode to direct access on exercise!

Leg Swings (No. 44)

Objective: Warm up and increase the mobility of the hips and legs, improve circulation, and prepare muscles and joints for more intense exercises.

STEP 1: Place one hand on a stable support.

STEP 2: Slightly lift the heel of the opposite foot.

STEP 3: Swing the free leg back and forth, keeping the torso still.

STEP 4: Repeat 5 times on each side.

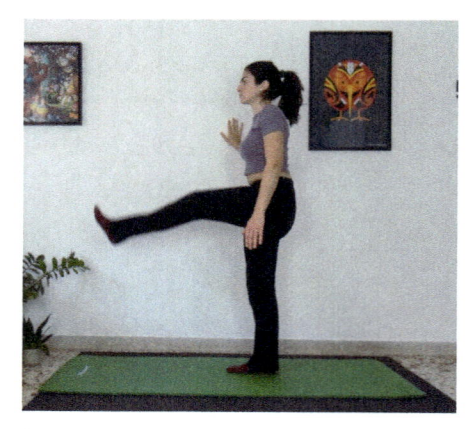

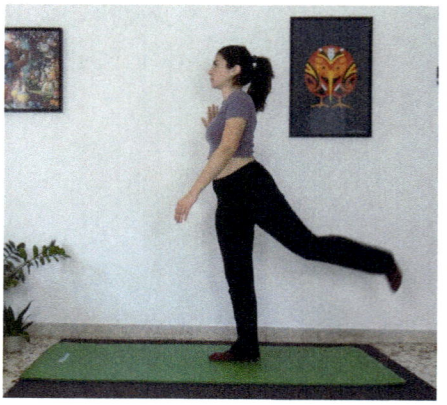

Cat-Cow Stretch (No. 45)

Objective: Improve the flexibility and mobility of the spine, while also helping to relax the mind and body.

STEP 1: Start on all fours, hands under shoulders, knees under hips. Neck aligned and gaze at the floor.

STEP 2: "Cat": Inhale, push the pelvis up, belly down, head and tailbone up.

STEP 3: "Cow": Exhale, pelvis down, arch the back, head down.

STEP 4: Repeat 4 times.

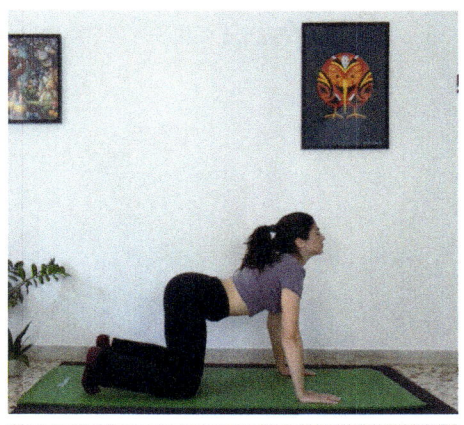

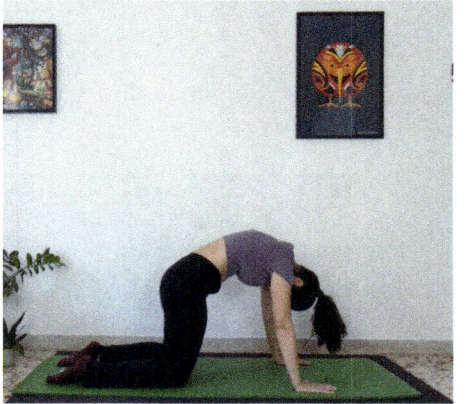

Scan this QRcode to direct access on exercise!

Ankle Circles (No. 46)

Objective: Improve the mobility and circulation of the ankles, preventing injuries and preparing the joints for movements that require stability and agility.

STEP 1: Sit on a chair, maintaining an upright posture.

STEP 2: Lift one foot and rotate the ankle: 5 circles clockwise, then 5 counterclockwise.

STEP 3: Repeat with the other ankle.

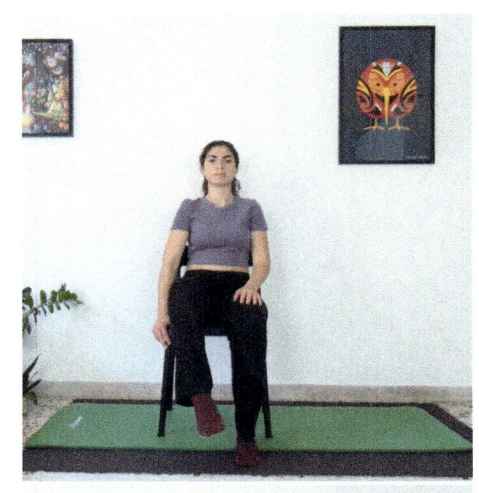

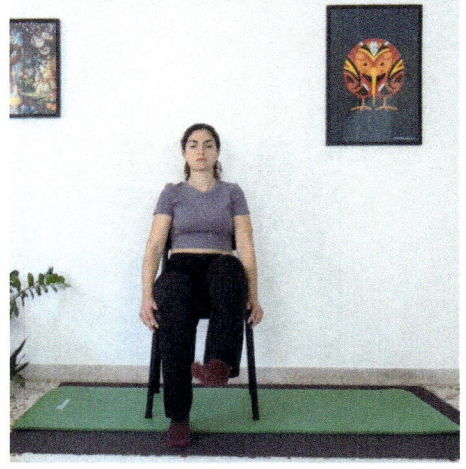

Dynamic Pigeon Pose (No. 47)

Objective: *Improve the flexibility of the hips and glutes, relieving tension and stiffness, particularly useful for those who spend many hours sitting.*

Scan this QRcode to direct access on exercise!

STEP 1: Start on all fours.

STEP 2: Bring your right leg forward, bending the knee, positioning the foot near the opposite knee.

STEP 3: Keep your back straight and chest lifted, stretching the right hip.

STEP 4: Return to all fours and repeat 3 times on each side, alternating.

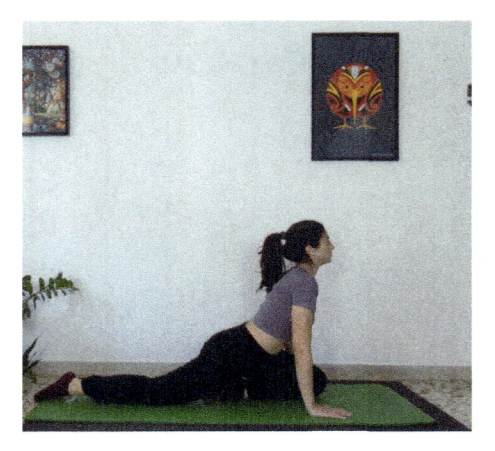

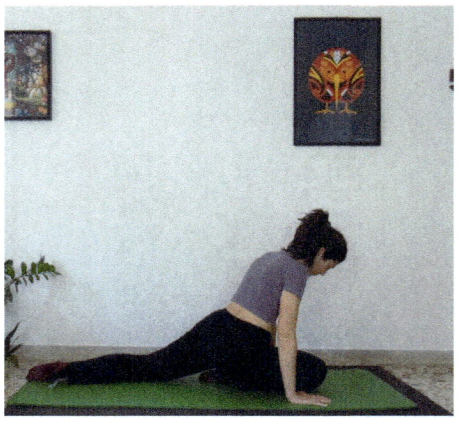

Pelvic Tilts (No. 48)

Objective: *Relieve tension in the lower back, improving pelvic mobility.*

STEP 1: Lie on your back with knees bent and feet flat on the floor.

STEP 2: Flatten your back against the floor by contracting your abdominal muscles and tilting your pelvis upward.

STEP 3: Relax your muscles and return to the starting position. Repeat 10 times.

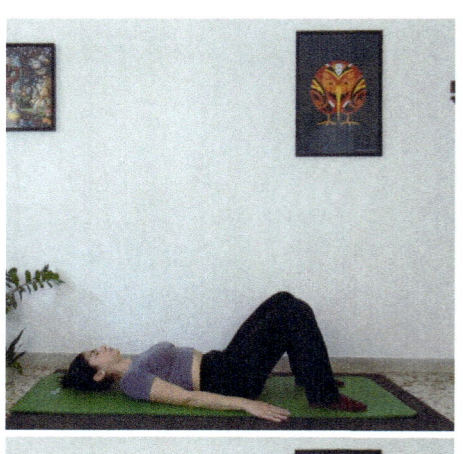

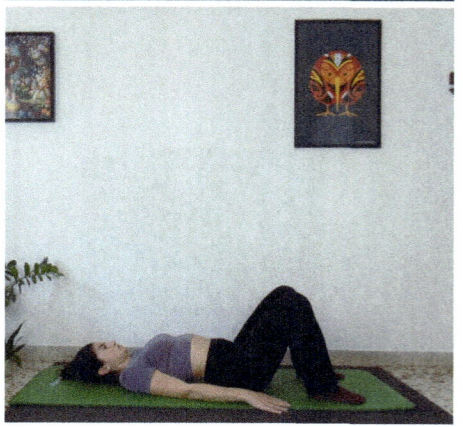

Butterfly Stretch (No. 49)

Objective: Increase flexibility in the groin and hips, improving joint mobility.

STEP 1: Sit on the floor with the soles of your feet together and knees opened out to the sides.

STEP 2: Hold your feet with your hands and gently press your knees down repeatedly, simulating butterfly wings for 20-30 seconds. Repeat 2-3 times.

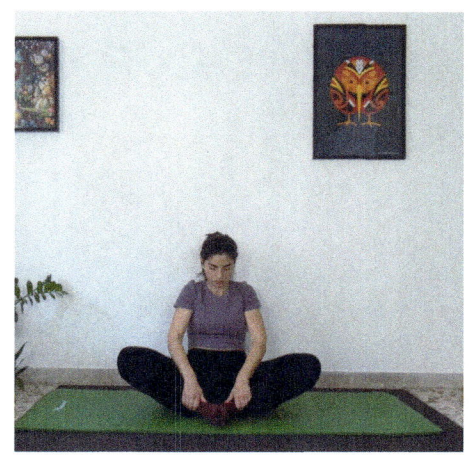

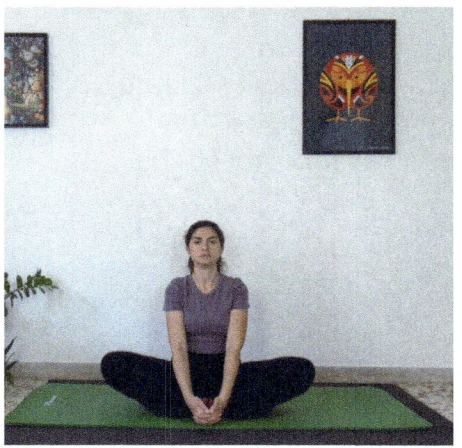

Scan this QRcode to direct access on exercise!

Neck Side Stretch (No. 50)

Objective: Reduce tension in the neck and improve lateral neck flexibility.

STEP 1: Sit or stand with your back straight.

STEP 2: Gently tilt your head toward one shoulder, bringing your ear toward the shoulder without lifting the shoulder.

STEP 3: Hold the position for 10-15 seconds, then switch sides and repeat.

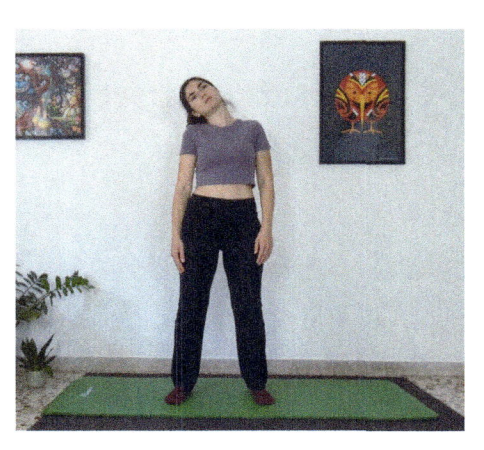

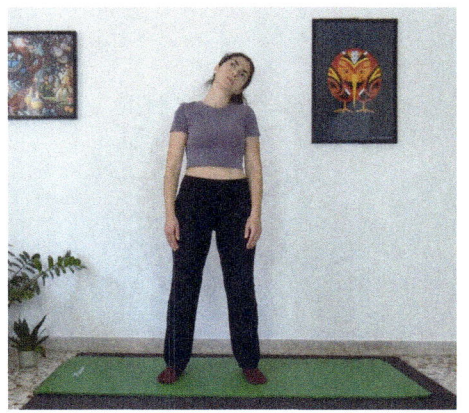

Shoulder Stretch with a Stick (No. 51)

Objective: Relieve tension in the shoulder muscles and upper chest, increasing shoulder flexibility and improving posture.

Scan this QRcode to direct access on exercise!

STEP 1: Stand or sit, holding a stick with both hands behind your back, keeping it horizontal.

STEP 2: Lift your arms as much as possible, keeping the stick steady between your hands. Ensure your arms are fully extended without arching your back or raising your shoulders.

STEP 3: Hold the position for 10 seconds, feeling a stretch along your shoulders and chest. Release slowly and repeat 2 times.

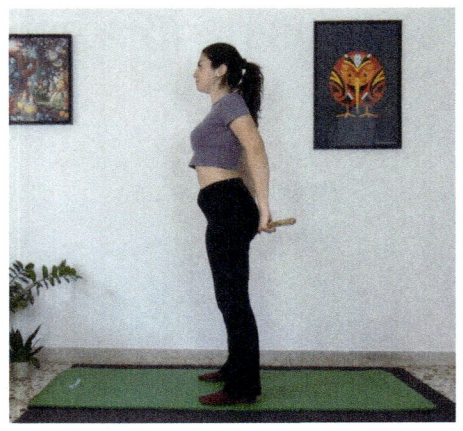

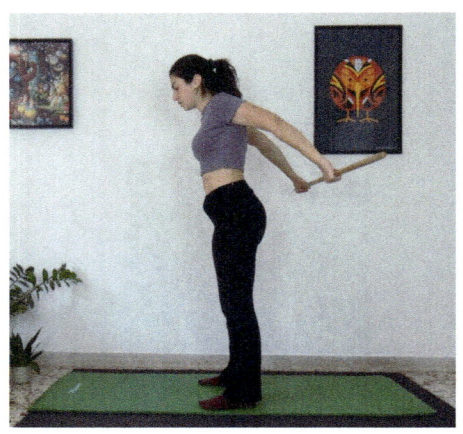

Seated Hamstring Stretch (No. 52)

Objective: Increase the flexibility of the hamstrings, improving the mobility of the back of the thigh.

STEP 1: Sit on the floor with one leg extended and the other bent so that the foot touches the inner thigh of the opposite leg.

STEP 2: Lean your torso forward from the hip toward the extended leg, trying to reach your foot with your hands.

STEP 3: Hold the position for 20 seconds and switch legs. Repeat 2-3 times per leg.

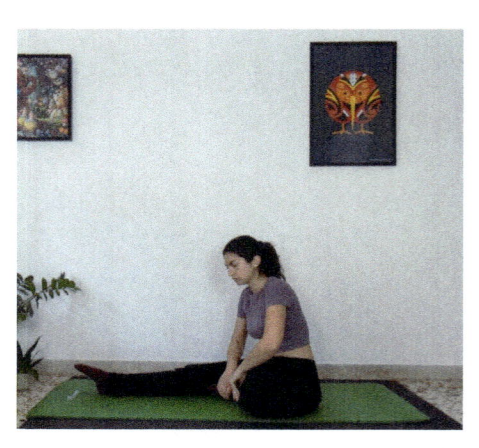

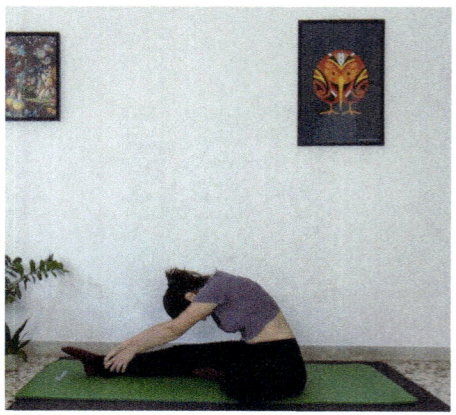

4.2 Muscle Awakening Exercises

Marching On Place (No. 53)

Objective: Warm up the leg joints and increase heart rate.

STEP 1: Stand with feet shoulder-width apart, arms at your sides.

STEP 2: Alternate lifting knees and opposite arms.

STEP 3: Maintain an upright posture and steady rhythm for 1 minute, breathing regularly to warm up the legs and increase heart rate.

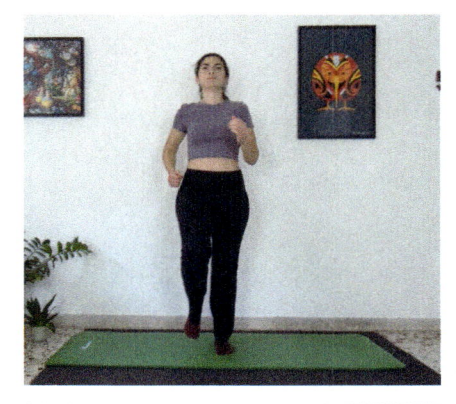

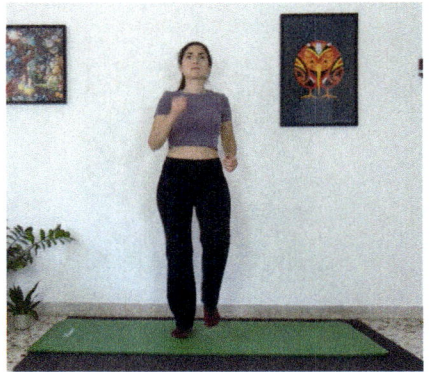

Scan this QRcode to direct access on exercise!

Arm Circles (No. 54)

Objective: Improve circulation and shoulder mobility, warming up and preparing the muscles of the arms and back for more intense activities.

STEP 1: Stand with feet shoulder-width apart, back straight, shoulders relaxed.

STEP 2: Raise your arms laterally to shoulder height.

STEP 3: Make 8 large circles, first forward then backward.

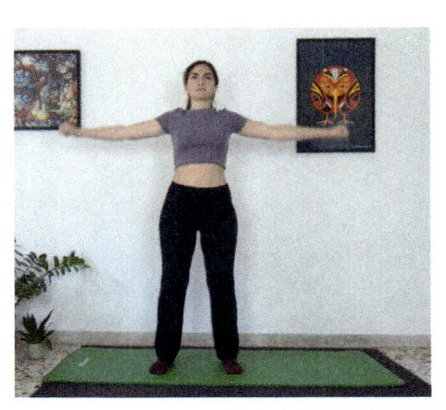

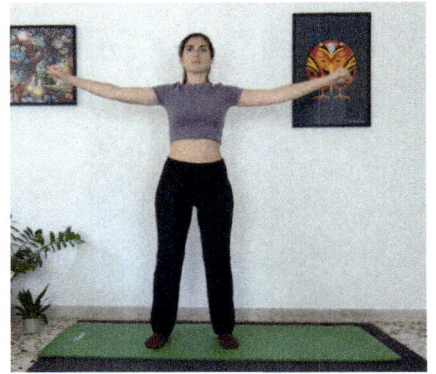

Jumping Jacks (No. 55)

Objective: Increase heart rate, warm up the whole body, and improve coordination and overall mobility.

Scan this QRcode to direct access on exercise!

STEP 1: Stand with feet together.

STEP 2: Jump, spreading your feet beyond shoulder width and raising your arms above your head.

STEP 3: Return to the starting position and repeat 10 times.

Intermediate: 15 reps
Advanced: 20 reps

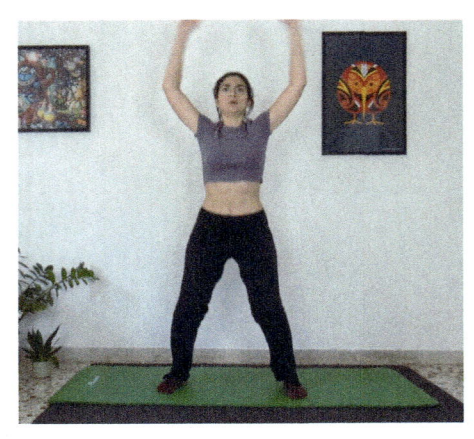

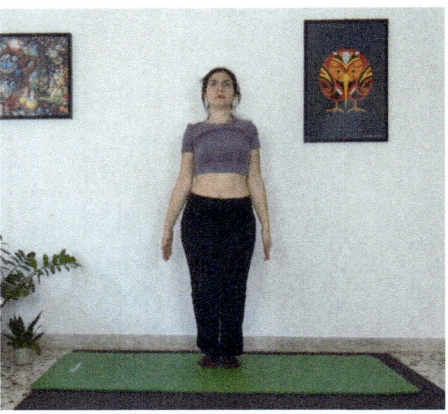

High Knees (No. 56)

Objective: Improve leg coordination and mobility while strengthening core muscles.

STEP 1: Stand with feet shoulder-width apart, chin up.

STEP 2: Rapidly alternate lifting knees toward the chest.

STEP 3: Maintain a steady and accelerated rhythm for 15 seconds, ensuring an upright posture. Focus on contracting the abdominal muscles while lifting the knees toward the chest.

Intermediate: 20 sec.
Advanced: 25 sec.

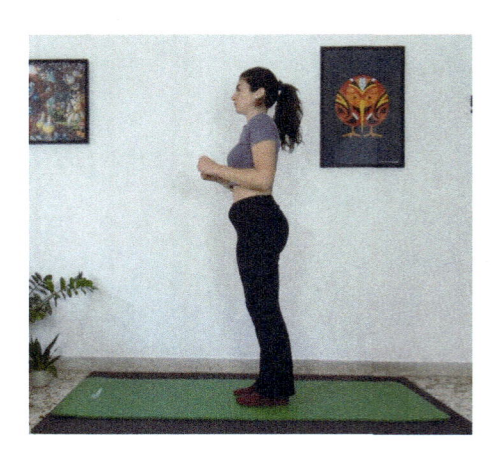

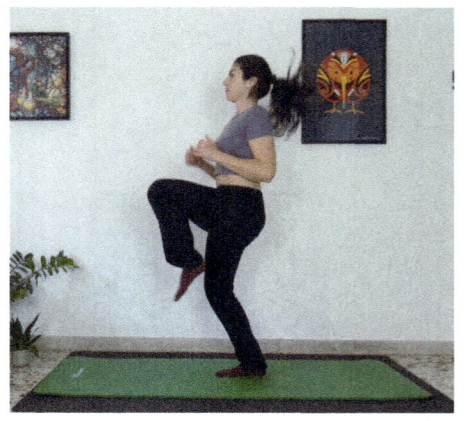

Inchworms (No. 57)

Objective: Increase core strength and spinal flexibility, improving stability and preparing the body for bodyweight or weight exercises..

Scan this QRcode to direct access on exercise!

STEP 1: Start standing, bend the torso forward and touch the floor with your hands, keeping your legs straight.

STEP 2: "Walk" your hands forward until you reach a plank position, keeping your core engaged and shoulders over wrists.

STEP 3: Return to the starting position by "walking" your hands back to your feet and slowly standing up, head last.

STEP 4: Repeat 2 times.

Intermediate: 4 reps
Advanced: 6 reps

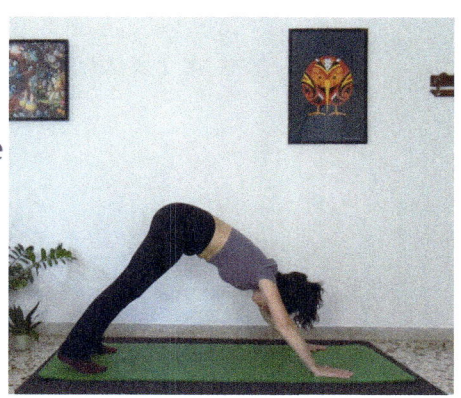

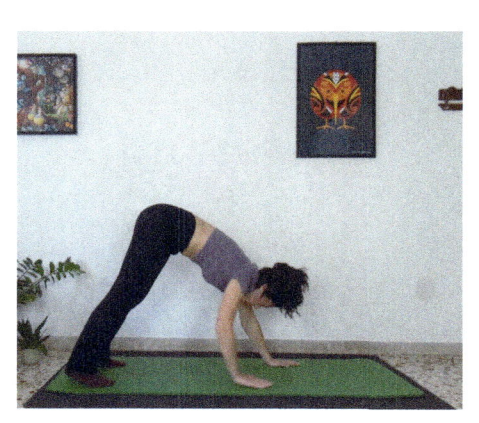

Butt Kicks (No. 58)

Objective: Increase heart rate and improve quadriceps flexibility.

STEP 1: Start standing with feet shoulder-width apart.

STEP 2: Run in place, bringing your heels towards your glutes as quickly as possible.

STEP 3: Continue "kicking" your glutes with your heels for 30 seconds x 2 sets.

Intermediate: 45 sec. x 2 sets
Advanced: 1 min x 3 sets

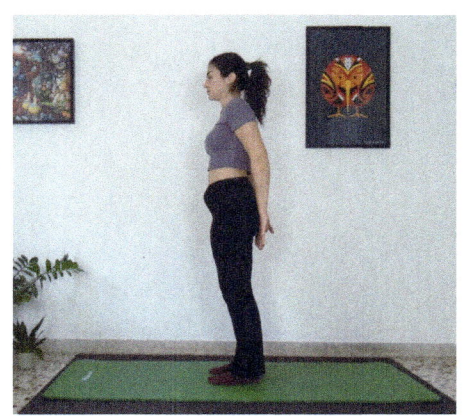

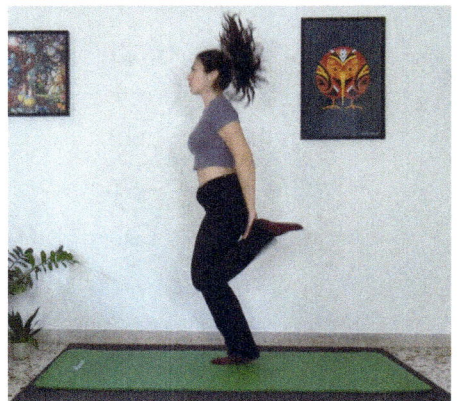

Bear Crawl (No. 59)

Objective: *Improve core strength, coordination, and overall stability.*

Scan this QRcode to direct access on exercise!

STEP 1: Get on all fours with knees slightly lifted off the ground.

STEP 2: Move forward by alternating the opposite movement of arms and legs, keeping your back flat.

STEP 3: Continue moving forward for 10 meters, then back, x 2 sets.

Intermediate: 2 sets x 15 meters
Advanced: 3 sets x 20 meters

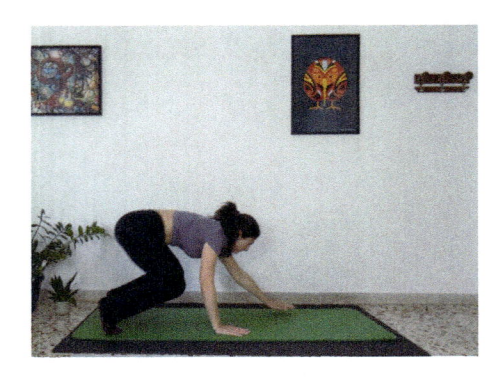

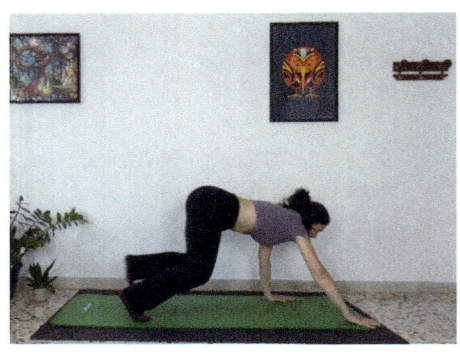

Slide and Glide (No. 60)

Objective: *Increase agility and fluidity of lateral movement, improving coordination and balance.*

STEP 1: Stand with feet together.

STEP 2: Slide laterally, shifting weight onto the leading foot, then bring the other foot along in a smooth and controlled motion.

STEP 3: Repeat the movement to the opposite side in a continuous and rhythmic motion.

Beginner: 30 sec. x 2 sets
Intermediate: 45 sec. x 3 sets
Advanced: 60 sec. x 3 sets

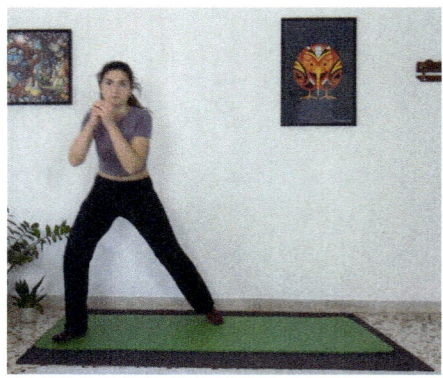

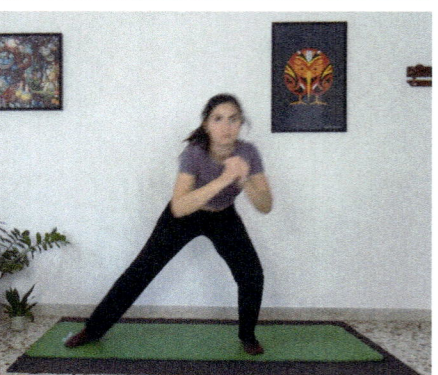

Boxer Shuffle (No. 61)

Objective: Increase heart rate and improve agility.

STEP 1: Stand with feet slightly apart and raise your arms.

STEP 2: Quickly shift your weight from one foot to the other, maintaining a fast pace.

STEP 3: Simulate boxing with your arms simultaneously for 30 seconds x 2 sets.

Intermediate: 45 sec. x 3 sets
Advanced: 1 min x 4 sets

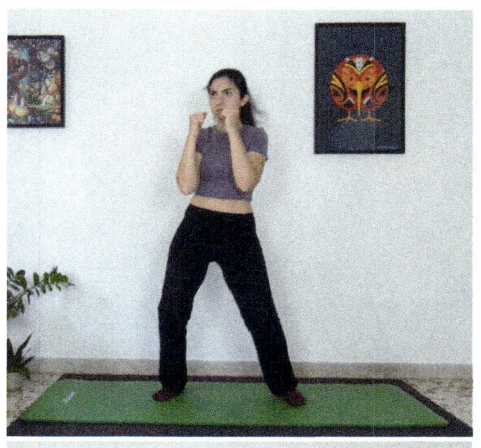

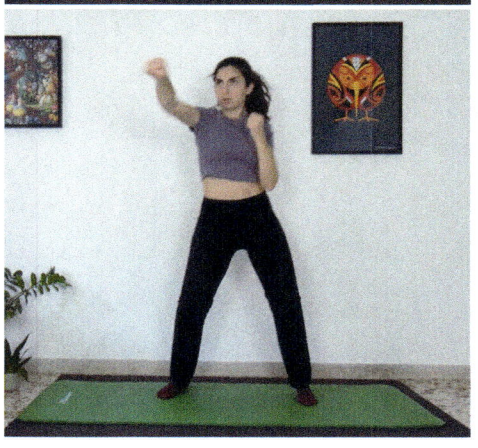

Scan this QRcode to direct access on exercise!

Knee Lifts (No. 62)

Objective: Improve core strength and leg mobility.

STEP 1: Stand with feet shoulder-width apart.

STEP 2: Lift your right knee towards your chest, then lower it and repeat with the left knee.

STEP 3: Continue alternately lifting knees for 30 seconds x 2 sets.

Intermediate: 45 sec. x 2 sets
Advanced: 1 min x 3 sets

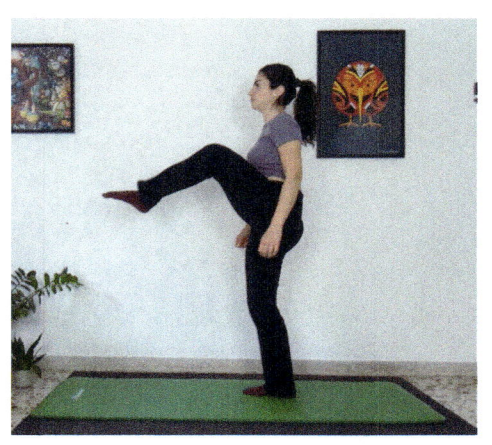

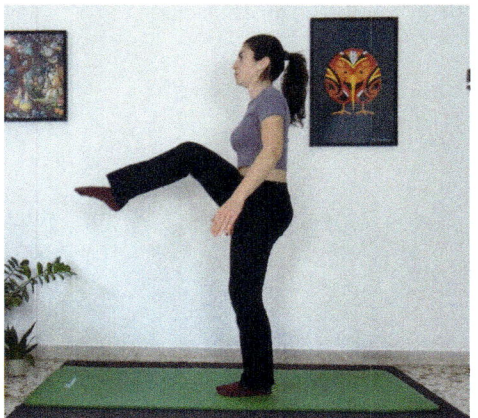

Chapter 5: Muscle Strengthening Exercises

5.1 Basic Muscle Strengthening Exercises

Core Exercises

Modified Plank (No. 63)

Objective: Strengthen core muscles, improving stability and posture, suitable for those seeking a less intense version of the traditional plank.

Scan this QRcode to direct access on exercise!

STEP 1: Start on all fours.

STEP 2: Lower your elbows to the floor and lift your knees off the ground, bringing your body into a straight line from head to feet.

STEP 3: Hold the position for 15-20 seconds and repeat 2 times with 1 minute of rest.

Intermediate: 30 sec. x 2 sets
Advanced: 45 sec. x 2 sets

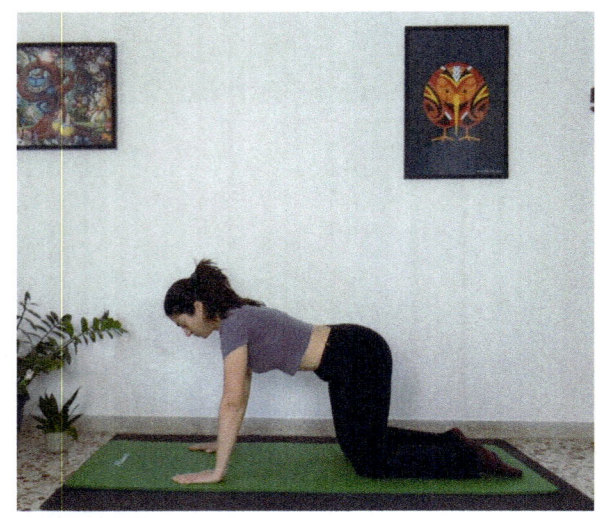

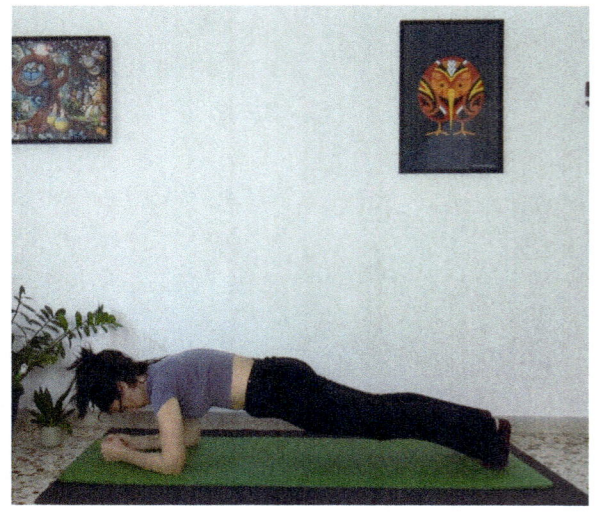

Core Exercises

Modified Crunch (No. 64)

Objective: Increase abdominal strength with less impact on the back compared to traditional crunches.

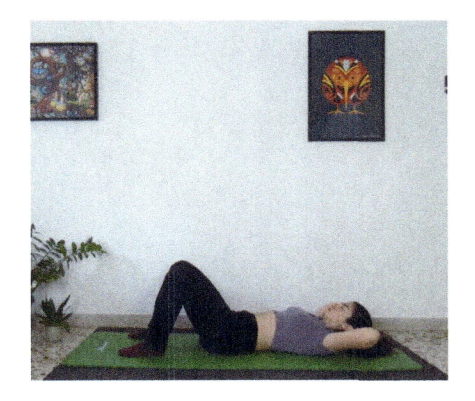

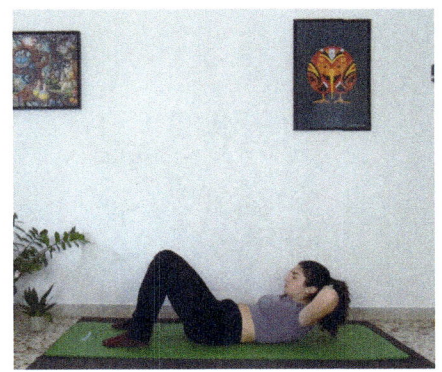

Scan this QRcode to direct access on exercise!

STEP 1: Lie on your back with knees bent and feet flat on the floor.

STEP 2: Lift your head and shoulders off the floor; keep your feet fixed.

STEP 3: Slowly return to the starting position.

STEP 4: Perform 10 repetitions for 2 sets.

Intermediate: 12 reps x 2 sets
Advanced: 15 reps x 3 sets

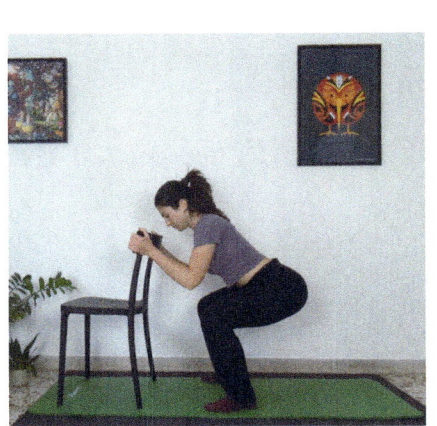

Basic Leg Exercises

Assisted Squat (No. 65)

Objective: Improve leg and glute strength, and hip and knee joint mobility, using a chair for support and safety.

STEP 1: Stand facing a chair for support.

STEP 2: Perform a squat, keeping your heels on the ground until your hips are parallel to the floor.

STEP 3: 8 repetitions for 2 sets.

Intermediate: 12 reps x 2 sets
Advanced: 15 reps x 2 sets

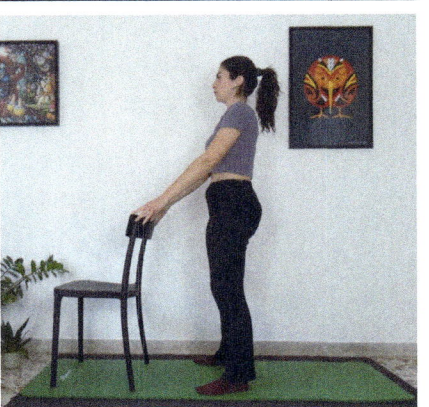

Basic Leg Exercises

Static Lunges (No. 66)

Objective: Increase strength and stability in the leg and glute muscles by maintaining a fixed position.

STEP 1: Step forward with one leg.

STEP 2: Bend both knees to 90 degrees, hold the position for a few seconds, then step back.

STEP 3: 8 repetitions per leg for 2 sets.

Intermediate: 10 reps per leg x 2 sets
Advanced: 12 reps per leg x 3 sets

Scan this QRcode to direct access on exercise!

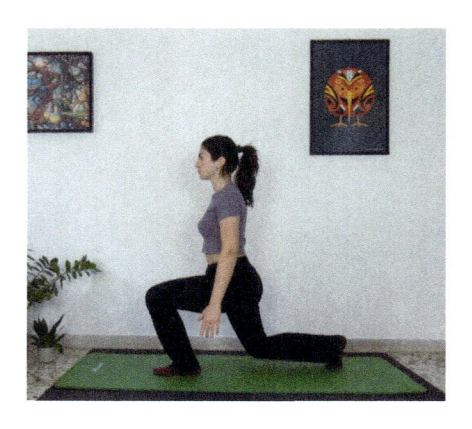

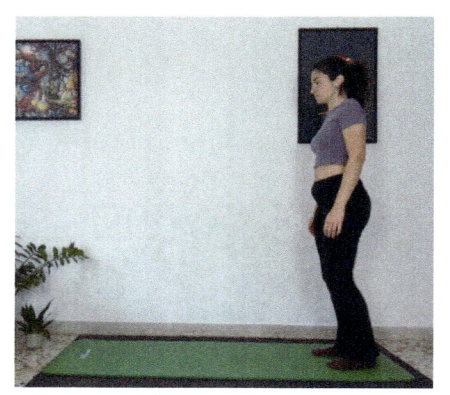

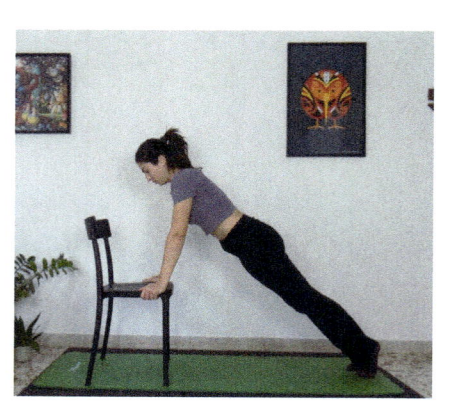

Arm Strengthening Exercises

Modified Push-up (No. 67)

Objective: Strengthen the chest, shoulders, and triceps with a more accessible version of the classic push-up.

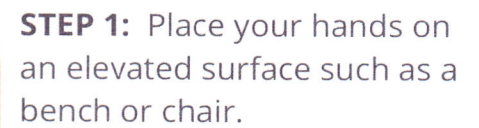

STEP 1: Place your hands on an elevated surface such as a bench or chair.

STEP 2: Bend your elbows to 90 degrees, lowering your body, then fully extend your arms.

STEP 3: 4 repetitions for 2 sets.

Intermediate: 8 reps x 2 sets
Advanced: 10 reps x 2 sets

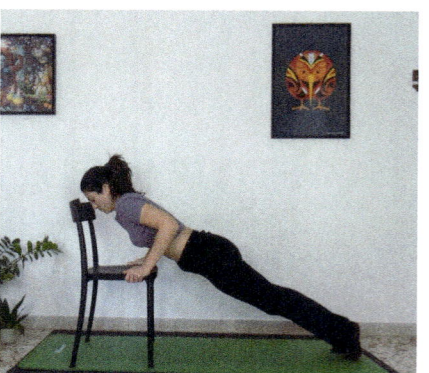

Arm Strengthening Exercises

Water Bottle Curl (No. 68)

Objective: Increase bicep strength and improve arm-hand coordination using a water bottle as a light weight.

STEP 1: Stand, holding a water bottle in each hand.

STEP 2: Bend your elbows, bringing the bottles toward your shoulders, then lower slowly.

STEP 3: 8-10 repetitions per arm for 2 sets.

Intermediate: 10 reps x 3 sets
Advanced: 15 reps x 3 sets

Scan this QRcode to direct access on exercise!

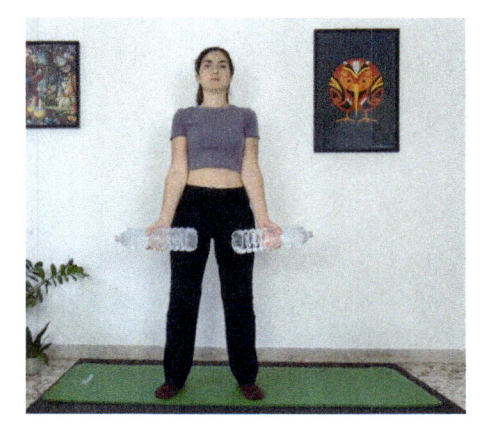

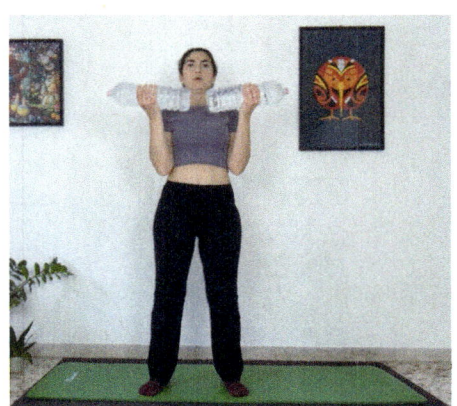

5.2 Functional Exercises for Everyday Activities

These exercises can be easily performed at home. They are great for people of all ages, especially those looking to maintain or improve their ability to perform daily tasks safely and efficiently.

Movements That Simulate Daily Activities

Loading and Unloading a Box (No. 69)

Objective: Simulate moving objects.

STEP 1: Bend your knees into a squat, lift a box from the floor to your chest.

STEP 2: Place it on a shelf and repeat to return it to the floor.

STEP 3: 8-10 repetitions.

Intermediate: 12 reps
Advanced: 15 reps

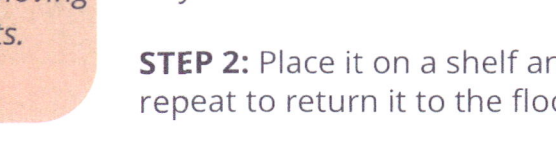

Scan this QRcode to direct access on exercise!

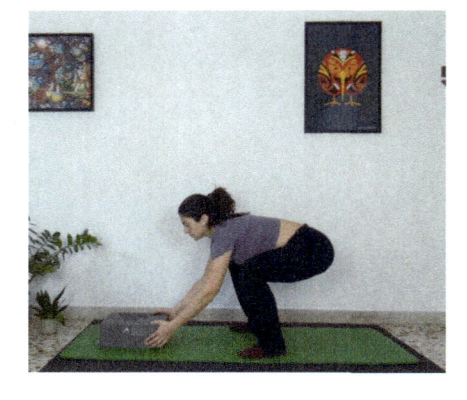

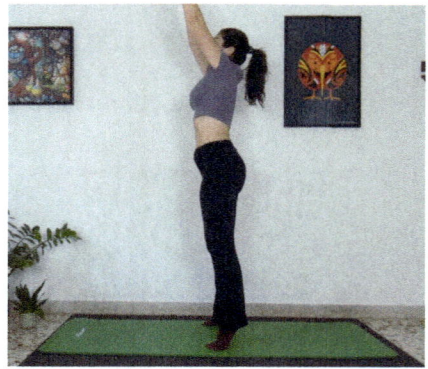

Walking with Weights (No. 70)

Objective: Simulate carrying groceries.

STEP 1: Hold a weight in each hand.

STEP 2: Keep the weights steady at your sides for 2 minutes.

Intermediate: 3 min
Advanced: 4 min

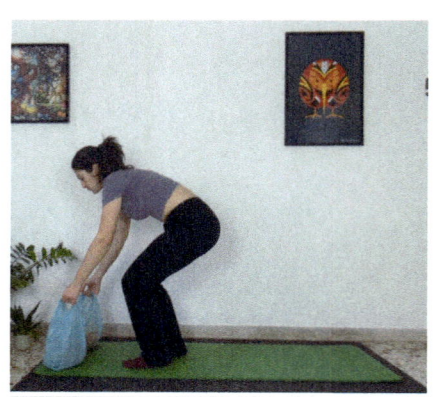

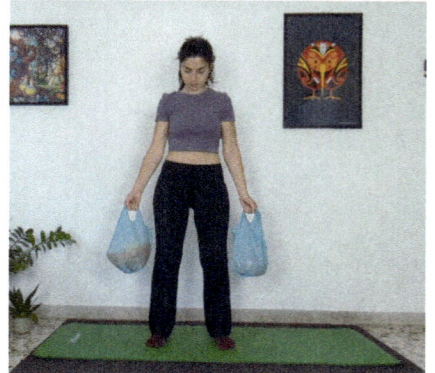

Exercises to Improve Balance and Prevent Falls

Single Leg Raises (No. 71)

Objective: Simulate putting on pants while standing.

Scan this QRcode to direct access on exercise!

STEP 1: Stand, lift one foot off the ground, maintaining balance on the other foot.

STEP 2: Hold the position for at least 10 seconds, then switch feet.

Intermediate: 15 sec.
Advanced: 20 sec.

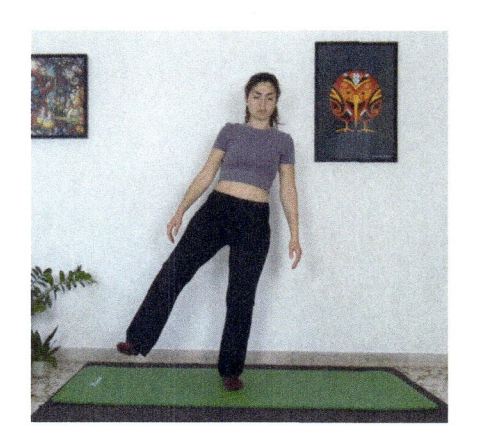

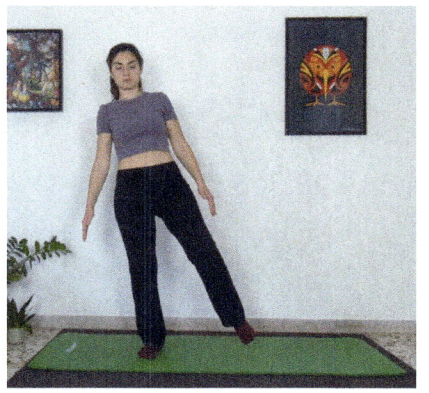

Side Foot Tap (No. 72)

Objective: Simulate bending laterally to pick up objects from the floor without rotating the body. Develop balance and proprioception.

STEP 1: Stand with arms at your sides, move one foot to the side, lightly touching the floor, and return to the starting position.

STEP 2: Repeat 10 times per side.

Intermediate: 15 reps per side
Advanced: 20 reps per side

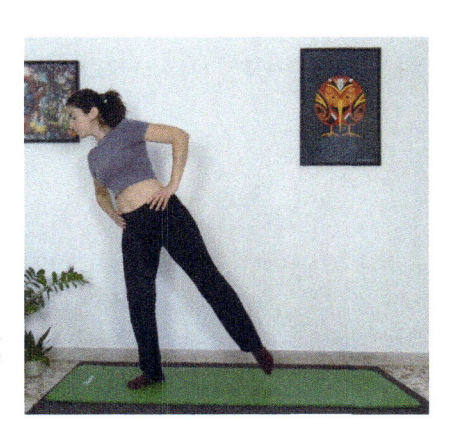

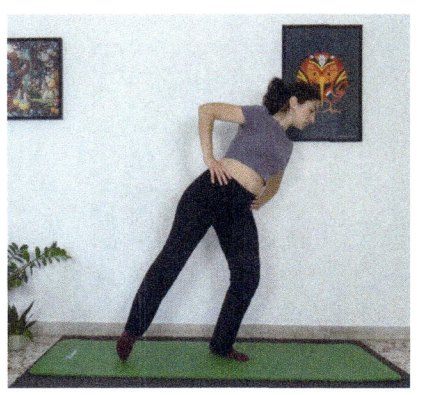

Techniques to Improve Coordination and Responsiveness

Slalom with Cones (No. 73)

Objective: Simulate quick movements and changes in direction.

STEP 1: Set up small objects on the ground as markers and, starting from one side, zigzag between them as quickly as possible.

STEP 2: Repeat the course 3-5 times.

Intermediate: 8 reps
Advanced: 12 reps

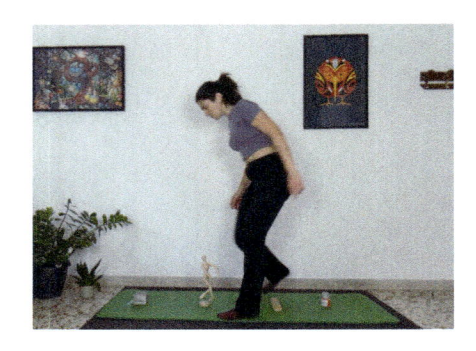

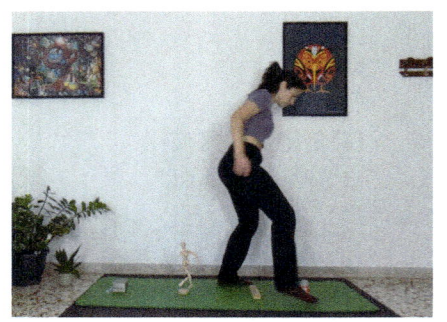

Scan this QRcode to direct access on exercise!

Overball and Wall (No. 74)

Objective: Improve hand-eye coordination.

STEP 1: Standing about 1.5 meters from the wall, throw an overball against the wall and catch it on the rebound. (Throw and catch with both hands.)

STEP 2: Perform 10-12 throws.

Intermediate: 15 throws
Advanced: 18 throws

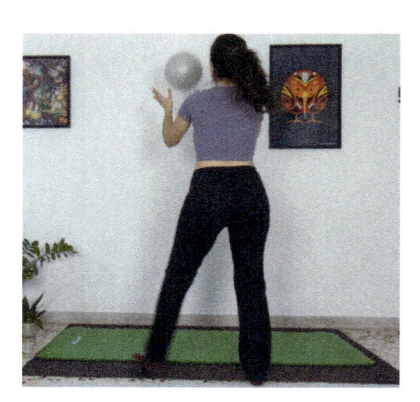

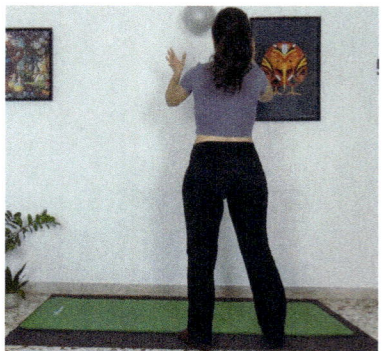

5.3 Integration of Small Equipment

Using Bands and Small Weights

Lateral Raises with Band (No. 75)

Objective: Strengthen the shoulder and back muscles, improving scapular mobility and stability, useful for preventing shoulder pain and injury.

Equipment: Pilates band -
Beginners: soft
Intermediate: semi-hard
Advanced: hard

STEP 1: Stand with the band under your feet, holding the ends with your hands, arms at your sides.

STEP 2: Raise your arms laterally to shoulder height, then lower them in a controlled manner.

STEP 3: 8-10 repetitions for 2 sets.

Scan this QRcode to direct access on exercise!

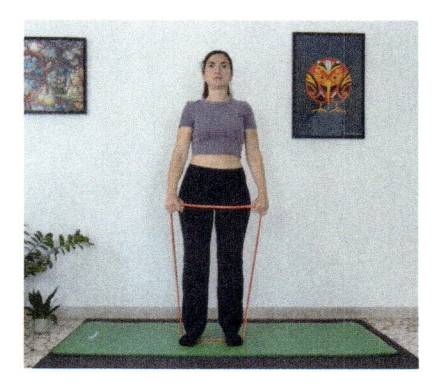

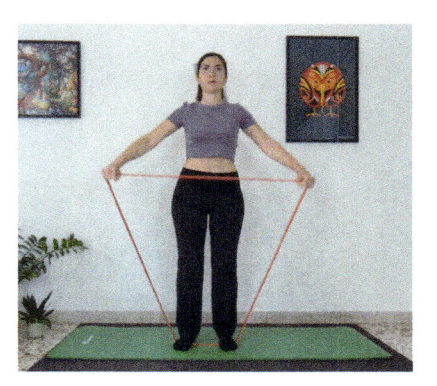

Front Extensions with Small Weights (No. 76)

Objective: Increase strength in the front arm muscles, particularly the biceps and deltoids, promoting better muscle definition and endurance.

Equipment: Dumbbells -
Beginners: 2 kg
Intermediate: 3 kg
Advanced: 4 kg

STEP 1: Stand or sit with back straight, holding a weight in each hand.

STEP 2: Raise straight arms to shoulder height, then lower them slowly.

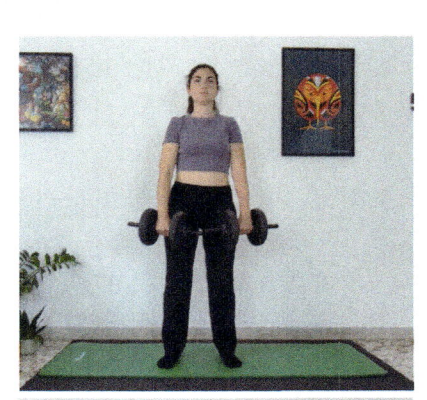

STEP 3: 8-10 repetitions for 2 sets.

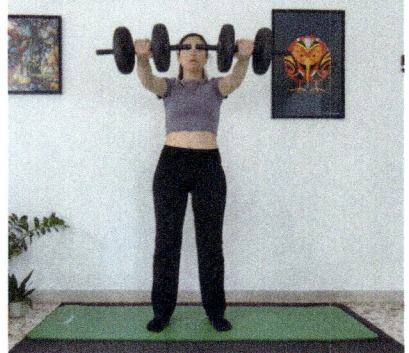

Exercises with a Tennis Ball

Foot Massage (No. 77)

Objective: Improve blood circulation in the feet, relieve tension and pain, and promote a general sense of relaxation.

STEP 1: Stand or sit on a chair, place a tennis ball under one foot.

STEP 2: Press and move the foot on the ball back and forth for 1-2 minutes per foot.

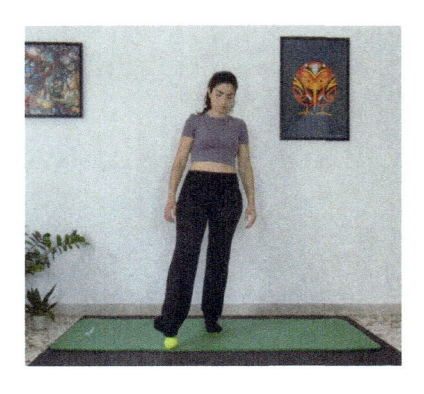

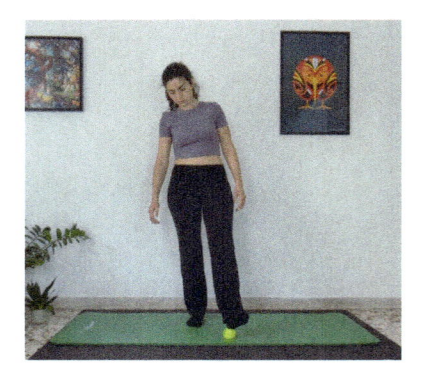

Scan this QRcode to direct access on exercise!

Trapezius Relaxation (No. 78)

Objective: Reduce muscle tension and pain in the trapezius muscles, common areas of stress accumulation, improving posture and reducing the risk of headaches and neck pain.

STEP 1: Stand with shoulders against a wall, place a tennis ball on the muscle between the shoulder blade and spine.

STEP 2: Press your body against the ball and make small movements, vertical and horizontal, to massage the trapezius for 1-2 minutes per side.

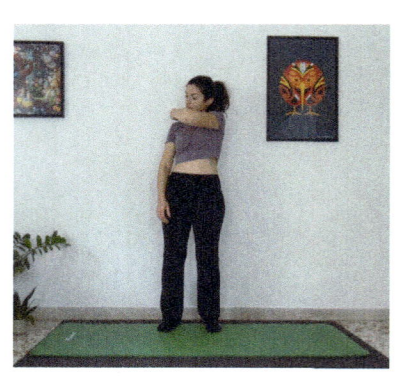

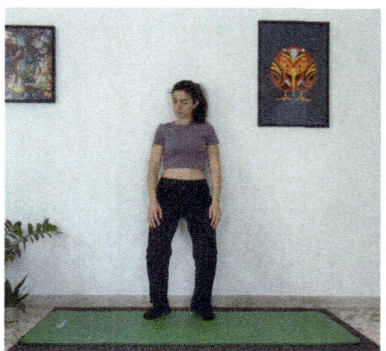

Exercises with a Overball

Overball Squat (No. 79)

Objective: *Strengthen leg and core muscles, maintaining balance and coordination. The Overball adds instability that further stimulates stabilizer muscles.*

STEP 1: Stand, holding a Overball between your knees.

STEP 2: Perform a squat, keeping the Overball steady.

STEP 3: 10-12 repetitions for 2 sets.

Intermediate: 12 reps x 3 sets
Advanced: 15 reps x 3 sets

Scan this QRcode to direct access on exercise!

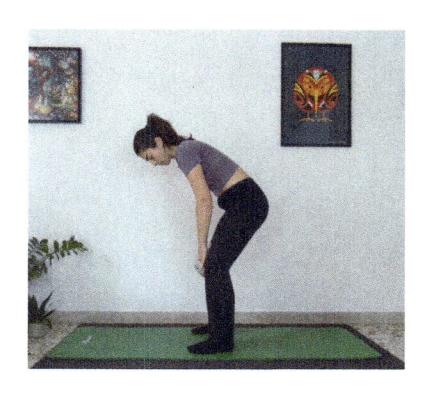

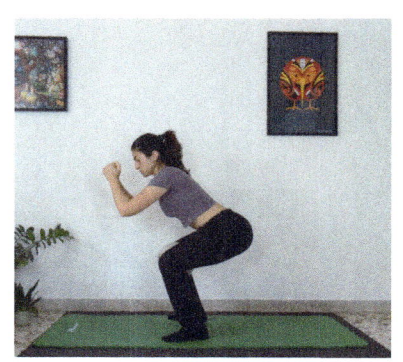

Overball Back Extensions (No. 80)

Objective: *Improve strength and flexibility of the spine, helping to prevent back pain and improving overall posture.*

STEP 1: Lie face down, with the Overball under your stomach.

STEP 2: Slowly lift and lower your chest, keeping the Overball stable.

STEP 3: 8-10 repetitions for 2 sets.

Intermediate: 10 reps x 3 sets
Advanced: 15 reps x 3 sets

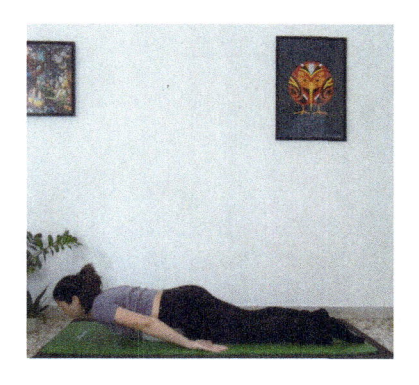

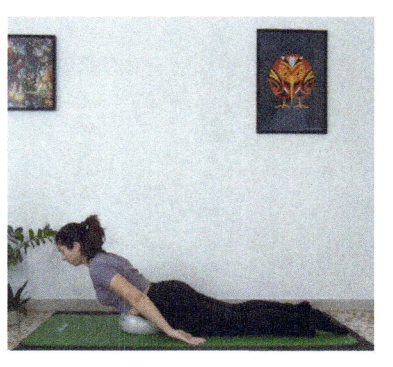

5.4 Weight Loss Exercises

Jump Squats (No. 81)

Objective: Burn calories and increase leg power.

Scan this QRcode to direct access on exercise!

STEP 1: Start standing with feet shoulder-width apart.

STEP 2: Perform a squat, then jump explosively.

STEP 3: Land softly in a squat position and repeat.

Intermediate: 15 reps x 3 sets
Advanced: 20 reps x 3 sets

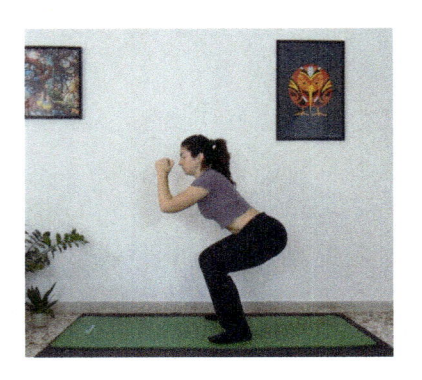

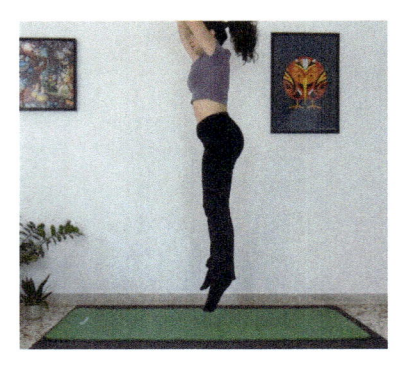

Burpees (No. 82)

Objective: Increase heart rate and work multiple muscle groups simultaneously.

STEP 1: Start standing.

STEP 2: Lower into a squat, place hands on the ground, and jump back into a plank position.

STEP 3: Return to the squat position and jump up with arms raised. Repeat x 5 times.

Intermediate: 10 reps x 2 sets
Advanced: 15 reps x 3 sets

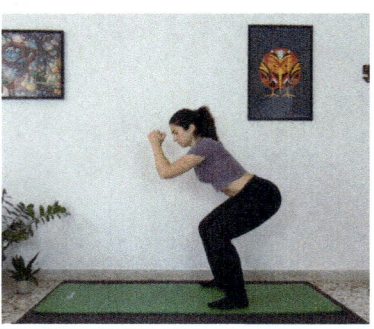

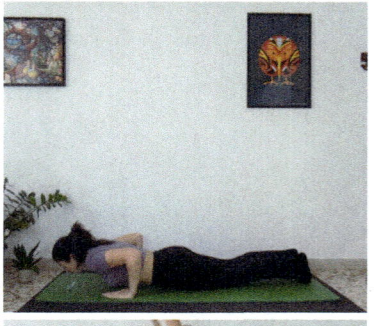

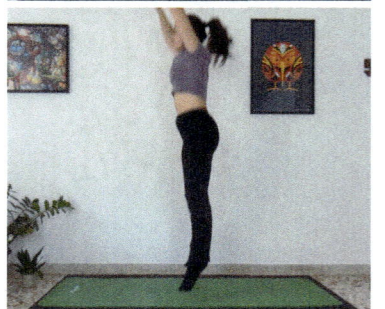

Mountain Climbers (No. 83)

Objective: Improve cardiovascular endurance and tone the core.

Scan this QRcode to direct access on exercise!

STEP 1: Start in a plank position.

STEP 2: Quickly bring one knee towards the chest, then alternate with the other.

STEP 3: Continue rapidly alternating legs.

Intermediate: 30 sec x 3 sets
Advanced: 45 sec x 3 sets

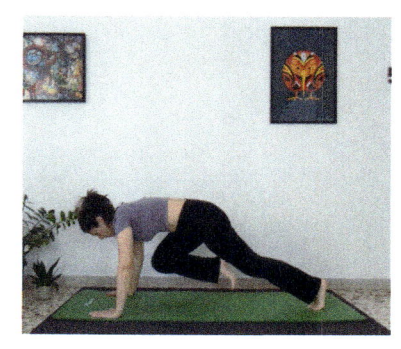

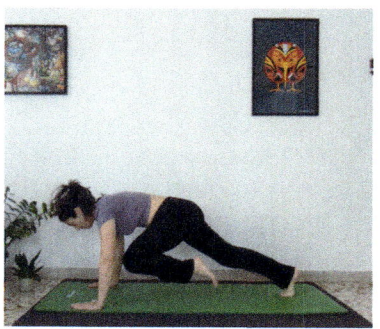

Side Plank (No. 84)

Objective: Strengthen oblique muscles and improve lateral core stability.

STEP 1: Start lying on one side, propping up on one elbow, with elbow under the shoulder and legs extended.

STEP 2: Lift hips off the floor creating a straight line from head to feet.

STEP 3: Hold the position for 15-20 seconds then switch sides.

Beginner: 15 sec. x 2 sets per side
Intermediate: 30 sec. x 2 sets per side
Advanced: 45 sec. x 2 sets per side

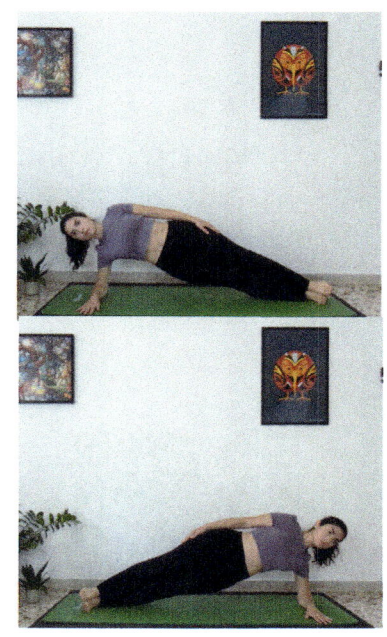

Moderate Reverse Crunch (No. 85)

Objective: Strengthen lower abdominal muscles and improve core stability.

STEP 1: Lie on your back with hands at your sides or under your glutes for support.

STEP 2: Lift bent legs toward the chest, contracting your abs.

STEP 3: Slowly lower legs without touching the floor and repeat.

Beginner: 10 reps x 2 sets
Intermediate: 15 reps x 2 sets
Advanced: 20 reps x 3 sets

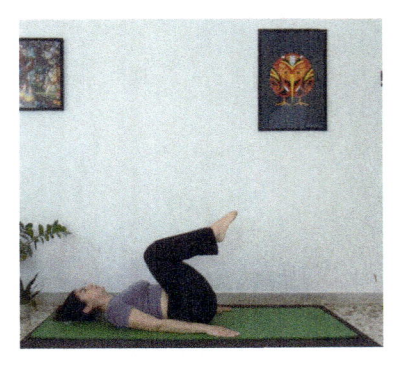

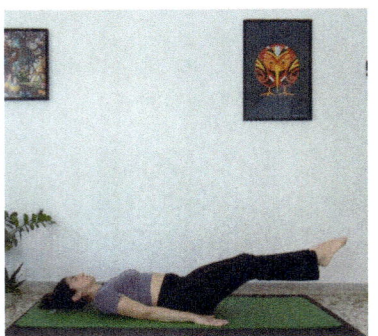

Scan this QRcode to direct access on exercise!

Speed Skaters (No. 86)

Objective: Increase lateral endurance and leg power.

STEP 1: Start standing with legs slightly apart.

STEP 2: Take a large step sideways to the left, bringing the right foot behind you, lightly touching the floor.

STEP 3: Quickly alternate sides.

Intermediate: 20 sec x 3 sets
Advanced: 30 sec x 3 sets

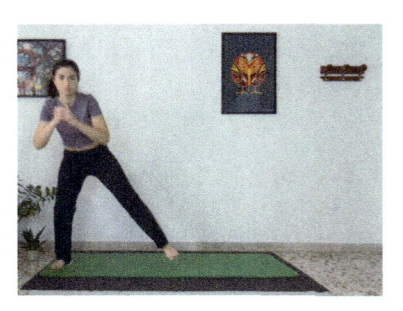

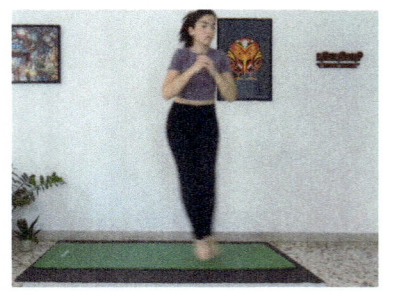

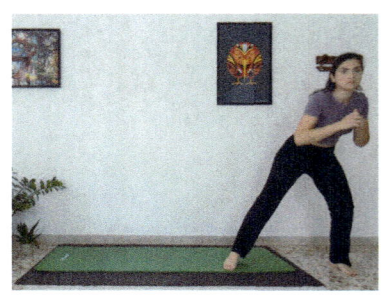

Superman Exercise (No. 87)

Objective: Strengthen lower back muscles and core, improving spinal stability.

STEP 1: Lie face down with arms extended in front of you and legs straight.

STEP 2: Simultaneously lift arms and legs off the ground as if flying like Superman. Ensure to lift using back muscles, not the neck.

STEP 3: Hold the elevated position for 3 seconds then return to starting position. Repeat x 2 sets with 1 minute rest.

Intermediate: 15 sec. x 2 sets - 1 min. rest
Advanced: 20 sec. x 3 sets - 1 min. rest

Scan this QRcode to direct access on exercise!

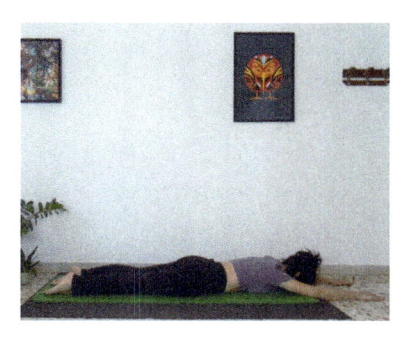

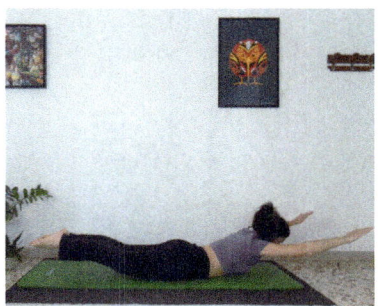

Plank to Downward Dog (No. 88)

Objective: Improve core strength and overall body flexibility.

STEP 1: Start in plank position on hands and feet.

STEP 2: Push hips back toward the ceiling, transitioning to downward dog pose, keeping arms and legs straight.

STEP 3: Return to plank position and repeat 5 cycles x 2 sets with 1 min. rest.

Intermediate: 8 cycles x 2 sets with 45 sec. rest
Advanced: 10 cycles x 3 sets with 30 sec. rest

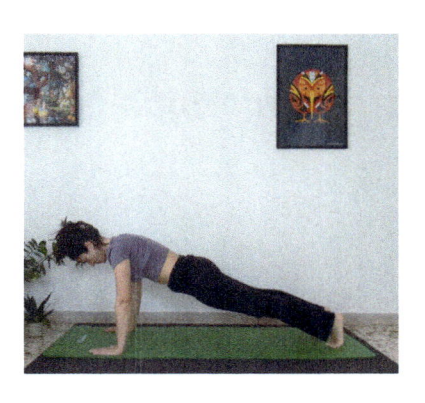

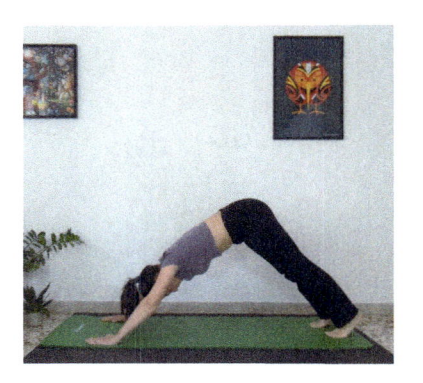

Push-Ups with Rotation (No. 89)

Objective: Strengthen core and upper body strength.

Scan this QRcode to direct access on exercise!

STEP 1: Start in a modified plank on knees, with hands under shoulders and body straight from head to knees.

STEP 2: Perform a push-up, lowering chest close to the floor, keeping core engaged.

STEP 3: Return to modified plank, lift one arm and rotate torso upward, extending the arm toward the ceiling. Look toward the raised hand and maintain balance. Perform 4 reps x 2 sets with 1 min. rest.

Intermediate: 6 reps x 3 sets - 45 sec. rest
Advanced: 10 reps x 4 sets - 30 sec. rest

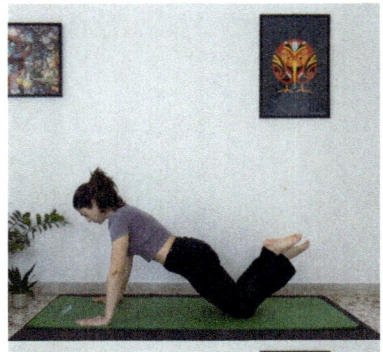

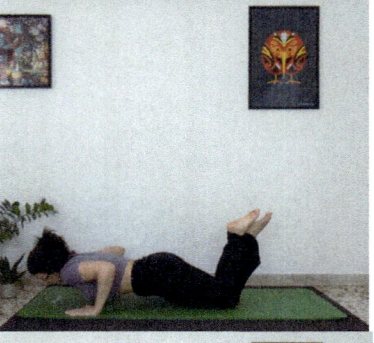

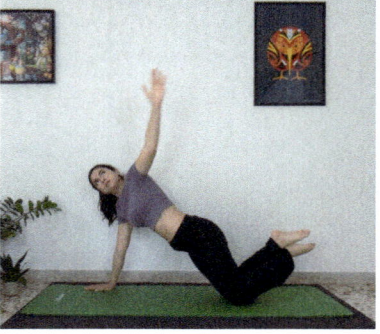

Spiderman Plank (No. 90)

Objective: Improve core and leg mobility, strengthen upper body muscles, and enhance core stability.

STEP 1: Lower into a plank position, with hands placed directly under shoulders.

STEP 2: Bring the right knee towards the right elbow, then return to plank position and repeat 4 times per side x 2 sets.

Intermediate: 6 reps per side x 2 sets
Advanced: 8 reps per side x 3 sets

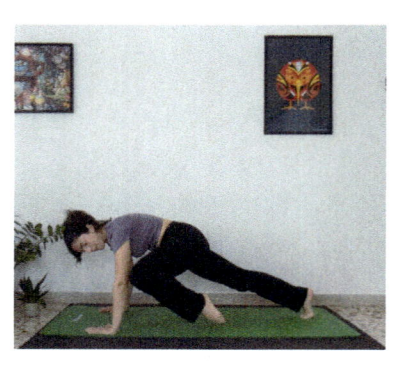

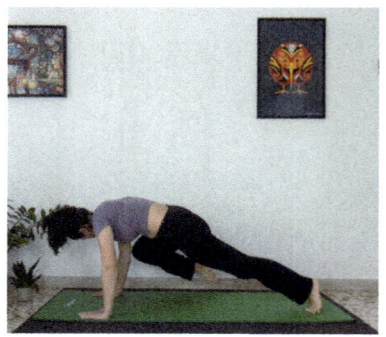

Chapter 6: 28-Days Challenge

It's crucial to recognize the signals your body sends, indicating you are ready to move from the beginner level to intermediate, and subsequently, to advanced. Here's how you can identify the right moment to make these transitions.

From Beginner to Intermediate Level:
Consolidation of Basics: First and foremost, you should feel completely comfortable with the basic exercises. This means being able to perform them with good form, without excessive fatigue.

Increased Ease: If you start noticing that the current exercises are no longer as challenging as they once were, and you can complete them easily without feeling particularly tired, it's a signal that your body has adapted and you can increase the difficulty.

Desire for More Challenges: Listen to your body and mind. If you feel the urge to explore exercises that require more coordination, strength, or endurance, it's probably time to move to the next level.

Physical Results: If your initial goals, such as improved mobility, reduced pain, or increased strength, have been achieved, it might be time to set new goals and challenges.

From Intermediate to Advanced Level:
Mastery of Intermediate Exercises: You should be able to perform all intermediate exercises with ease and precision. Mastery indicates that your body is ready for even more complex and intense exercises.

No Visible Progress: If after a period of consistent training, you no longer see improvements or changes, your body might have fully adapted to the intermediate level. It's time to introduce new challenges to stimulate progress.

Body and Mind Feedback: Your energy level, motivation, and desire to try more difficult exercises are key indicators that you are ready to advance to the next level. Listen to your physical and mental sensations.

Continuous Monitoring: Keeping a workout diary to track your progress can help you decide when it's the right time to advance. Record how often exercises become easier and your fatigue level after each session.

At every stage of your journey with somatic exercises, it's crucial to proceed with caution and awareness, always respecting your body's limits. Progression should be a conscious decision, based on both your personal feelings and the advice of qualified fitness professionals.
   Enjoy your advancement in your path towards somatic well-being!

Preparations before starting the challenge:

- Ensure to perform the exercises with correct technique and maximum intensity.

- **Warm up** for 5-10 minutes before beginning each workout session (follow the exercises outlined in subsection 4.1 of the book);

- The repetitions provided are for each set of exercises;

- The number of sets increases as the fitness level progresses;

- Always **listen** to your body and stop exercises if you experience excessive pain or discomfort.

- The **goal** of the challenge is to lose weight and regain overall physical, mental agility and **well-being**.

Week/Day	Jump Squats (81)	Mountain Climbers (83)	Push-Ups with Rotation (89)	Reverse Crunch (85)	Series	Rest Time (sec)
Beginner						
Week 1 Mon. - Sat.	10-12	10-12	5-7	8-10	2	60
Week 2 Mon. - Sat.	10-12	12-15	7-9	10-12	2	60
Week 3 Mon. - Sat.	12-15	15-18	9-11	12-15	2	60
Week 4 Mon. - Sat.	15-20	18-20	11-13	15-20	2	60
Intermediate						
Week 1 Mon. - Sat.	10-12	12-15	7-9	10-12	3	45
Week 2 Mon. - Sat.	12-15	15-18	9-11	12-15	3	45
Week 3 Mon. - Sat.	15-18	18-20	11-13	15-18	3	45
Week 4 Mon. - Sat.	18-20	20-25	13-15	18-20	3	45
Advanced						
Week 1 Mon. - Sat.	12-15	15-18	9-11	12-15	4	30
Week 2 Mon. - Sat.	15-18	18-20	11-13	15-18	4	30
Week 3 Mon. - Sat.	18-20	20-25	13-15	18-20	4	30
Week 4 Mon. - Sat.	20-25	25-30	15-18	20-25	4	30

Conclusion

We have reached the end of our journey, and I hope you have found this book to be both a **helpful** guide and an **encouraging** resource to start and maintain a **somatic exercise practice** that not only improves mobility and reduces accumulated stress but also enhances body awareness and overall **well-being**.

Through the various exercises presented, you have learned how to move your body in ways that support joint **health**, muscle strength, and most importantly, **stress reduction**. Each exercise has been designed to be accessible, easy to perform, and safe, regardless of your initial fitness level.

Remember that **regular practice** is the key to reaping the maximum benefits from somatic movements. I encourage you to take time each day for yourself to practice, explore, and **connect** with your body. Like any new habit, the beginning might seem challenging, but with commitment and perseverance, the benefits will be long-lasting and **deeply transformative**.

If you found value in this book and would like to help others discover the benefits of somatic exercises, I would be **grateful** if you could take a moment to leave a **review** on Amazon.com. Your opinions and experiences can inspire and motivate others to embark on their journey toward somatic well-being.

Thank you for choosing to accompany me on this journey. Keep moving mindfully and living well. I hope you continue to explore and deepen your somatic practice and that these exercises become a valuable part of your daily routine.

With **gratitude**,

Sophia Harmon

BONUS

Below you will find the **3 BONUSES**, always available to you, which you can access by scanning the QR code with your smartphone!

Inside you will find:
- **20 FAQs** to help you clarify any uncertainties or doubts before, during, and after performing the somatic exercises;

[QR code]

- A **Checklist** to track your weekly progress, which you can print and fill out as often as you like;

[QR code]

- **Inspiring Testimonials** from people who, like you, were experiencing high levels of somatized stress and achieved exceptional results within a few weeks of incorporating somatic exercises into their routines. Read these testimonials when your motivation wanes; they will help keep it high :)

[QR code]

NOTE:

NOTE:

Printed in Great Britain
by Amazon